Concentric Space as a Life Principle beyond Schopenhauer, Nietzsche and Ricoeur

Concentric Space as a Life Principle beyond Schopenhauer, Nietzsche and Ricoeur invites a fresh vision of human experience and search for life meanings in terms of potential openings through relational space. Offering a radical spatial rereading of foundational ideas of the influential thinkers Schopenhauer, Nietzsche and Ricoeur, it argues that these ideas can be rethought for a more fundamental understanding of life, self and other.

This book offers a radical reconceptualisation of space as an animating principle for life through common, although previously hidden, features across the thought of Schopenhauer, Nietzsche and Ricoeur. It offers a fresh spatial interpretation of key themes in these thinkers' works, such as compassion, will to life, Dionysian rapture, will to power, selfovercoming, re-valuation of values, eternal recurrence, living metaphor and intersubjectivity. It proposes a spatial restructuring of experience from diametric spaces of exclusion towards concentric spaces of inclusion for an experiential restructuring towards unifying modes of experience. This spatial rereading of these major figures in philosophy directly challenges many previous understandings, to offer a distinctive spatial-phenomenological framework for examining a life principle.

This book will appeal to academics, researchers and postgraduates engaged in the study of philosophy, wellbeing, education and human development. The book's interdisciplinary scope ensures that it is also of interest for those in the fields of psychology, anthropology, psychoanalysis and culture studies.

Paul Downes is Associate Professor of Psychology, School of Human Development, Institute of Education, Dublin City University, Ireland. He has over 100 international peer-reviewed publications across areas of philosophy, psychology, education, law, anthropology and social policy and has given keynotes and invited presentations in 29 countries.

Concentric Space as a Life Principle beyond Schopenhauer, Nietzsche and Ricoeur

Inclusion of the Other

Paul Downes

Routledge
Taylor & Francis Group
LONDON AND NEW YORK

First published 2020
by Routledge
2 Park Square, Milton Park, Abingdon, Oxon OX14 4RN

and by Routledge
605 Third Avenue, New York, NY 10017

First issued in paperback 2021

Routledge is an imprint of the Taylor & Francis Group, an informa business

Publisher's Note
The publisher has gone to great lengths to ensure the quality of this reprint but points out that some imperfections in the original copies may be apparent.

British Library Cataloguing-in-Publication Data
A catalogue record for this book is available from the British Library

Library of Congress Cataloging-in-Publication Data
A catalog record has been requested for this book

Typeset in Bembo
by Taylor & Francis Books

ISBN 13: 978-1-03-208837-2 (pbk)
ISBN 13: 978-1-138-30693-6 (hbk)

For my wife, Aleksandra Jasniewicz, and our children, Eva and Michael Downes, with love

Contents

Figures

Acknowledgements

Chapter 3 builds on my article, Downes, P. (2017). Reconceptualising Schopenhauer's *Compassion* through diametric and concentric spatial structures of relation, *Enrahonar: An International Journal of Theoretical and Practical Reason*, 60, 81–98.

Chapter 9 is based on Downes, P. (2016). At the threshold of Ricoeur's concerns in *La Métaphore Vive*: a spatial discourse of diametric and concentric structures of relation building on Lévi-Strauss, *Ricoeur Studies/Etudes Ricoeuriennes*, 7 (2), 146–163.

Chapter 10 is based on Downes, P. (forthcoming, 2019). A living spatial movement of relation – reconceptualising key aspects of Ricoeur's *Oneself as Another* and Heidegger's *Being and Time, Ricoeur Studies/Etudes Ricoeuriennes*.

Abbreviations

Arthur Schopenhauer

FRP	*On the Fourfold Root of the Principle of Sufficient Reason and Other Writings*. Trans. D. E. Cartwright, E. E.Erdmann and C. Janaway. Cambridge: Cambridge University Press (1813/2012), Payne, NY: Dover Publications, Inc. (/1958).
MN	*Metaphysik der Natur: Herausgegeben und eingeleitet von Volker Spierling*, Philosophische Vorlesungen, Teil II. Munich, Zurich: Serie Piper (1984).
OBM	*On the Basis of Morality*. Trans. E. F. J. Payne. Providence, RI: Berghahn Books (1839/1995).
WN	*On the Will in Nature*. Trans. E. F. J. Payne. New York: Berg (1992).
WWRI	*The World as Will and Representation, Volume I*. Trans. J. Norman, A. Welchman and C. Janaway. Cambridge: Cambridge University Press (1859/2010).
WWRII	*The World as Will and Representation. Volume II*. Trans E. F. J. Payne.

Friedrich Nietzsche

BGE	*Beyond Good and Evil: Prelude to a Philosophy of the Future*. Trans. Helen Zimmern. New York: Dover Publications, Inc. (1997).
BT	*The Birth of Tragedy*. Trans. D. Smith. Oxford: Oxford University Press (1872/2000).
D	*Daybreak*. Trans. R. J. Hollingdale. Cambridge: Cambridge University Press (1881/1982).
EH	*Ecce Homo*. Trans. Duncan Large. Oxford: Oxford University Press (2007).
GM	*The Genealogy of Morals*. Trans. Horace B. Samuel. New York: Dover Publications Inc. (2003).

GS	*The Gay Science*. B. Williams (ed.). Trans. J. Nauckhoff and A. del Caro. Cambridge: Cambridge University Press (2001).
HH	*Human, All Too Human*. M. Faber (ed.). London: Penguin (1878/1994).
WP	*Will to Power*. Trans. W. Kaufmann and R. J. Hollingdale; W. Kaufmann (ed.). New York: Vintage Books (1968).
Z	*Thus Spoke Zarathustra*. Trans. W. Kaufmann. New York: Viking (1883–5/1954).

Paul Ricoeur

HHS	*Hermeneutics and the Human Sciences*. Trans. J. B. Thompson. New York: Cambridge University Press (1981).
MV	*La Métaphore Vive. The Rule of Metaphor: Multi-disciplinary Studies of the Creation of Meaning in Language*. Trans. R. Czerny, with K. McLoughlin and J. Costello. London: Routledge (1978).
OA	*Oneself as Another*. Chicago, IL: University of Chicago Press (1994).

Chapter 1

Introduction

A protolanguage of space as concentric and diametric space

The question of a veil of space must be identified and opened to engage with a life force, so that space is no longer a sterile medium for experience and thought. Habits of space need to be exposed to interrogate the ripples of space invading conceptual foundations of a life principle.

There is a spatial system of relations, a primordial spatial discourse pertaining to life that is embedded in the seminal works of Schopenhauer, Nietzsche and Ricoeur – and yet overlooked by each of them. All three thinkers invoke a prior spatial discourse implicitly in their works. Like Wordsworth, who crossed the Alps without realising it, they have opened the door to a prior level of understanding. However, they have not directly walked through these gateways. Passing through the frames of these doors brings with it a reverberation, a movement that rustles the foundations of each of these thinkers' works so that the prior spatial discourse opens up their texts, unsettles their basic assumptions and invites reconstruction of each of their understandings of a life principle.

This questioning involves space as a protolanguage – a protolanguage examined for illustrative purposes as imbued within basic concepts in the works of Schopenhauer, Nietzsche and Ricoeur, with implications for understanding inclusion of the Other and a life principle in spatial terms. The *question* of the vista of protolanguages that are not dependent on language was an implicit, albeit not primary, concern for both Nietzsche and Ricoeur.[1] Whereas Nietzsche's *Birth of tragedy* sought engagement with a universal prerepresentational language of music, purportedly prior to language through the Dionysian, Ricoeur's *Rule of metaphor* took a number of tentative steps towards uncovering a spatial system prior to language, akin to a protolanguage, although he did not take this further step. Similarly, key concepts of Schopenhauer regarding overcoming the boundaries of the *principium individuationis* to attain a prior mode of experience and his conception of compassion offer spatial understandings that can be construed as precursors to the proposed spatial protolanguage. A sustained argument for a protolanguage of space was not *directly* brought to the fore by any of these thinkers, although each offered works replete with spatial imagery.

A primordial prelinguistic spatial discourse, a protolanguage of space, as seeped itself into language but prior to language is being postulated in this book. Specific spatial systems of interaction are being argued to reside *not only within* language but as being also silently woven into fundamental concepts, in the assumption structure of key understandings of life and inclusion. This spatial questioning is not reducible to traditional issues such as space as an object or medium of perception, to space as an *a priori* category of understanding, to spatial metaphors and imagery in philosophical language or to a space for play of meaning *within* language.

Nietzsche seeks an inversion of Platonism, as one of his many reversals, to advocate for the primacy of the sensuous world over a supersensous world of Platonic ideal forms. This is resonant with Schopenhauer's commitment to the vitality of the body in his libidinal materialism. Likewise, with his emphasis on the flesh, Ricoeur's *Oneself as another* invokes a concept that challenges abstraction, while moving in the direction of the primacy of embodiment. Nietzsche not only reverses the supersensuous–sensuous diametric opposition; he puts into question the very assumptions of truth–illusion, reality–appearance for both realms, as he treats the aesthetic as being more primary than the true, even for the sensuous realm. For him, a truth of the sensuous is perspectival and constructed, while being beholden to a will to power prior to a will to truth. Yet Nietzsche's challenge to Platonic metaphysics has left him open to Heidegger's accusation that he is still locked within metaphysics as the last metaphysician. Reversing relationships within a diametric opposition still rests within the same structure.

Heidegger responds to Nietzsche,

> A path must be cleared for a new interpretation of the sensuous on the basis of a new hierarchy of the sensuous and nonsensuous. The new hierarchy does not simply wish to reverse matters within the old structural order, now reverencing the sensuous and scorning the nonsensuous. (Vol. I: 209)

Quite apart from issues of the nonsensuous as distinct from the supersensuous, and the need to go beyond hierarchy as such, Heidegger's vital point here is on the need to shift the very structure underlying the sensuous–nonsensuous diametric opposition: 'A new hierarchy and new valuation mean that the ordering *structure* must be changed' (Vol. I: 209, italics in original). Heidegger needed to go further to recognise that this change in the ordering assumption structure is a *spatial questioning*. Diametric opposition is not only a projected *structure*, it tends to be overlooked that diametric opposition is also a *space*.

A change to diametric opposition is a change to diametric space, to modify this diametric spatial structure into another spatial mode of relation. Moreover, this spatial questioning implicates a questioning of inclusion of the Other, inclusion of the counterpole (whether the relegated counterpole of the sensuous for Plato or the supersensuous for Nietzsche); a spatial-structural alternative is needed to a diametric exclusion and subservience of one pole to the hegemony of the Other. This questioning of conceptual foundations requires a protolanguage of space pertaining to movement from exclusion towards inclusion; it raises the question of a shift not only beyond binary oppositional thinking, but beyond diametric spatial thinking and diametric spatial *experience*.

Heidegger is quite dismissive of *spatial* concerns in Nietzsche: 'Viewed as a whole, Nietzsche's meditations on space and time are quite meagre. The few thoughts concerning time that inch beyond traditional notions are desultory' (Vol. II: 90). However, there is a need to challenge this view through analysing space at a different level of explanation in terms of the assumption structure of Nietzsche's seminal concepts. In doing so, an integrated structure for Nietzsche's seminal concepts can be found, in contrast to Heidegger's treatment of Nietzsche, which highlights structural concerns but not in terms of space: '[A]t the outset we are utterly unable to take up one single unequivocal anticipation of the articulated structure in which "eternal return", "will to power", and "revaluation of all values" would cohere as one, all of them with equal originality' (Vol. II: 168). The current argument is one that seeks to offer such an *integrated* structure – as a *spatial* structure – for these core dimensions of Nietzsche's thought, while commencing with interrogation of rapture as a major concern of Nietzsche in BT. Moreover, a spatial level of description is being postulated that is not merely reducible to space as subjective projection.[2]

An elision has taken place in the history of Western thought, an elision pertaining to space that runs conceptually prior to Platonic metaphysical assumptions of ideal forms in a realm of the supersensuous that gain primacy over the sensual world. This suppression of a spatial questioning, alongside a surreptitious reliance on spatial assumptions, needs to be brought to the fore. Space offers a relation prior to thingness, prior to the *reus* of the real. Is space not the most obvious mediator between the material and symbolic, the sensory and supersensory world? This obviousness has been additionally glossed over by a Cartesian prejudice that space is a nonentity, a merely static noninteractive phenomenon. Space needs to be seen as intimately entwined with a life principle. Interrogation of a life principle rarely tends to embrace the pulse of space.

The question of inclusion of the Other is not only a structural one but also a spatial one. It is fundamentally a question of restructuring the projection of us/them. This us/them structure frames understanding of the supposed norm versus the Other. The Other becomes a reification shorn of animation, a static category rendered passive and inert in this role as mere object of the gaze from the vantage point of the supposed norm. This process of Othering is prominently challenged by de Beauvoir in *The second sex* to critique a construct of 'woman' in terms of a male reference point as the norm. Similarly, Said's *Orientalism* offers an excoriating assault on Western projections onto Eastern cultures that construct the East as the Other; the other is dehumanized of lived experience, as a static lifeless exhibit in 'an imaginary museum without walls' (1978: 166). Like the construct of 'woman' as the second sex, Eastern cultures become defined abstractly in unitary terms of contrasts with a Western culture as norm. Both de Beauvoir and Said appeal to a background implicit life principle, through associating its excision with a principle of dynamic exclusion bringing 'the Other'; this exclusion renders concrete groups and individuals inert and lifeless, as abstract categories of the Other.

The exclusion process in the us/them projection rests on a diametric binary opposition, a projected *structure* of diametric *space*. For inclusion of the Other, as distinct from exclusion of the Other through diametric space, again a different space is needed, a space of difference, a structure of differential relation. This different space to foster connection with and inclusion of the other encompasses a different mode of experience, a different dimension of being. This different space is argued in this book to be one of concentric spatial relation.

An anthropological starting point for consideration of such spaces can move to a terrain far beyond the confines of subjectivism and anthropology, as well as beyond the epistemological commitments of Lévi-Strauss to a structuralist paradigm drawn from structural linguistics. Building on Lévi-Strauss' (1962, 1963, 1973) account of cross-cultural observations of these structures for myths and physical structures, a diametric spatial structure is one where a circle is split in half by a line that is its diameter, or where a square or rectangle is similarly divided into two equal halves (see Figure 1.1). In a concentric spatial structure, one circle is inscribed in another larger circle (or square); in pure form, the circles share a common central point (see Figure 1.2) – a co-centre.

Lévi-Strauss tended to treat these as structures rather than as spaces or fundamental modes of space.

A fundamental concern with *connection* pervades key concepts of both Schopenhauer and Ricoeur, whereas expansion of experience as *openness* and *reversal*

Figure 1.1 Diametric dualism

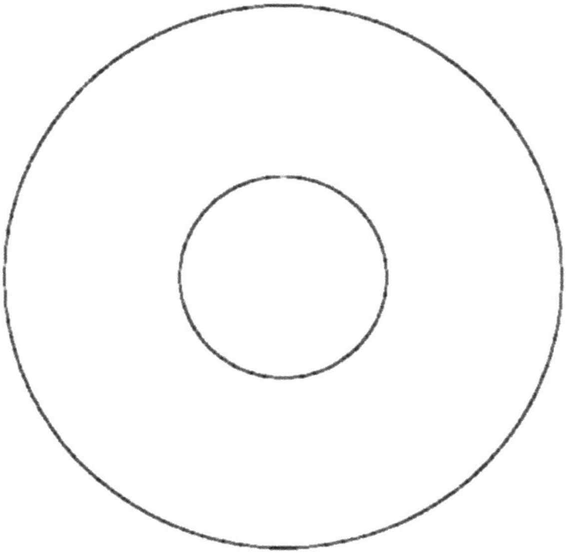

Figure 1.2 Concentric dualism

underpins a range of core concepts of Nietzsche. Connection and openness will be argued to be manifestations of distinct structures of experience in spatial terms – concentric space – with reversal a feature of diametric space. It will be argued that these seminal thinkers' basic concepts are held together through a common silent thread of space, not an inert space but the lost continent of an implicit spatial interplay between concentric and diametric spaces.

Schopenhauer's and Nietzsche's works are conceptually intertwined, with overt points of affinity and antagonism. Commonalities between these thinkers and Ricoeur are that they all invoke a life conception, at least implicitly, while also interrogating relations between self and another with regard to an axis of inclusion and exclusion. Each offers a challenge to the Cartesian ego, while giving emphasis to experience to challenge dry abstraction and simultaneously seeking also to move beyond the injunction of the Kantian categorical imperative, to act as you can at the same time will that it become a universal law. Significantly, each thinker silently relies on spatial assumptions for their understandings of life and experience. Ricoeur's particular contribution includes the proximity of his position to a spatial protolanguage and moreover, a spatial protolanguage integrally concerned with a life principle. Concern with inclusion of the Other is a key theme in his work. Kearney characterises Ricoeur as an 'inveterate mediator' (2007: 147) between traditions and positions; such a mediating role for Ricoeur can be taken further through recognition of the key role of space as a mediating dimension.

Space and a life principle

By lifeless space, it is meant space that is without movement, lacking not only animation but also being flattened into immateriality as abstraction. Descartes treated space as a lifeless nonentity, as a nothingness. A living space as a dynamic interacting background is in stark contrast with a Cartesian conception of space as 'empty' and a 'mere nonentity' (Descartes 1954: 200). It is this lifelessness for space that sets a foundation for lifeless space as abstraction. The question arises as to whether even those thinkers who offered a prolonged onslaught on abstraction, on a metaphysics beyond, such as Nietzsche, have overcome or even perceived this problem of lifeless space in their thought.

The shift that is needed for a conceptual movement in space, to apprehend a moving, life-giving space is one that treats thought as a material dimension[3] and hence is itself spatial. It attacks not merely disembodiment but the despatialisation into a flattened one- or two-dimensional space that has squeezed the life of breath out of space, out of even thought that seeks to animate life. This book seeks to remedy this despatialisation of thought as exemplified in Schopenhauer, Nietzsche and Ricoeur; this despatialisation has been the supporting condition to splinter thought from fundamental experiential projections – from proposed primordial experiential projections of concentric space and diametric space.

Moving space is the breath of thought. Yet space remains inert, flat and without this breath of movement in the foundations of Western thought. This problem of space is a blind spot even in the seminal thought of Nietzsche who did much to challenge the foundations of Western metaphysics and to rattle the cages of traditional assumptions. A breath-embodied thought is needed to address the dimensionality of space and to challenge a ferocious flattening of space. Spatial breath is the pulse of thought, not a denial of spatial breath in the inert space of monism. Space is indelibly interactive and immanent in thought. Even when space is not interacting with the objects of thoughts' constituents, this itself is revealing, as *noninteraction is itself a mode of interaction*.

As part of this unveiling of space, a thesis of this book is that there are limited structural options as projected grounds or horizons for fundamental conceptualisation. These are monism, diametric dualistic opposition and mirror image inverted symmetry (diametric space *simpliciter*), figure–ground as a variant of diametric spatial relations, and concentric space. These express implicit spatial structures of experience for the breath of thought.

These structures of monism, dualism etc. are not the metaphysics of an abstract beyond, a beyond that is fictive according to Nietzsche. These are the projections of spatial experience 'below', in our unconscious but not merely in a subjectivist sense. They are ineluctable tracks of our experiential preconditions framing thought. These are not isolated, random pockmarks projected into thought but a collective dynamic system, infused in our life experience of the breath. Monism is not simply a heuristic device for describing the organisation of concepts but a revealing spatial projection, as part of a system of potential projections of a range of spatial experiences.

The argument here is to set out the relevance of this spatial protolanguage rather than to offer proof that it is ineluctable for thought, it is a preliminary argument in this sense. The argument that space is an ineluctable feature of thought is not a simple argument that it is a transcendental condition as a necessity for thought (see Körner 1967 on the difficulty of *a priori* truth claims that need to rule out all possible hypothetical situations). For current purposes, an initial preliminary argument is being made that space, as a protolanguage, is a pervasive condition for thought pertaining to life understandings in basic concepts of Schopenhauer, Nietzsche and Ricoeur.

This spatial understanding turns metaphysics on its head. It does not claim some abstract supersensory reality above the physical; it does not proceed in diametric spatial terms into splits between the abstract–concrete, ideal–real, mind–body. Rather it seeks an accelerated immanence, one that is not mere reduction to the body or material. It is rather an engagement with space as a precondition for the body, as a precondition for the material and as embedded in experience, as a prior living precondition seeped into and through experience. Going further, it offers an interrogation of how these spatial projections become manifested in experience and thought, and treats thought as ineluctably spatial.

These framing spatial assumptions, while giving rise to infinite frameworks of thought and aspects of representational understanding, are themselves finite in structure and range. It is not necessarily being proposed that the range of primordial spatial projections uncovered and related to basic concepts in Schopenhauer, Nietzsche and Ricoeur's works are the only possible spatial ones. That is being left as an open question. However, it is being claimed that these possible spatial frames are a foundational and neglected 'deep' grammar of space, a language of space that is itself prior to language – a spatial protolanguage or discourse.

A spatial protolanguage can be reconstructed from thought assumptions, as dimensions of experience. Many previous frameworks postulating a protolanguage seek to derive this from more primitive ancient forms of language itself or from concepts or representations prior to language (Fitch 2010). A spatial protolanguage is being proposed as precognitive, prerepresentational; it is phenomenological through its ascribing primacy to the domain of experience as distinct from mind. Space is treated as a precondition for experience and language. Moreover, it offers a vantage point for the primordial that does not take the historical or the evolutionary as its starting point. It does not primarily seek to interrogate a spatial protolanguage within human prehistory. Rather, it interrogates the primordial in terms of prior epistemological and ontological assumptions, the assumption structure framing the conceptual; the referential concerns of truth as correspondence come later rather than being the starting point for inquiry.

A role for space in experience is being sought that is not simply that of serving as a diametric space of counterpole to the senses – of silence to sound, saliva to taste, background contours to define the shape of foreground object seen, of background air to fragrant smell and object touched. Space needs to emerge beyond the figure–ground variant of diametric space of assumed separation between mutually defining contrasts. Space is more than mere juxtaposition.

Space not only serves as such experiential content through a diametric function, but goes further as the very precondition for the senses to exist. Space shapes the senses more radically for experience; without it, the senses cease to exist, the *reus* of the thing is no longer real for experience. Space is a key governing condition for both reality and ideality, yet is subservient to neither, even as it is embedded in both. Concern is with the contours of this prior space, prior to the animism of the foreground–background interactions that govern the vitality of the senses. With a primordial spatial protolanguage, it is not a case of footprints imposed on the snow. It *is* the snow. It is the medium itself of experience.

In seeking to challenge Western metaphysics, thought itself must be rendered physical and hence spatial. There needs to be a selfreferential consistency between a content of thought that rejects the abstractions of metaphysics and the structure of thought that is thereby spatial and physical and not simply itself abstract. Parkes recognises this issue of different linguistic and conceptual levels in his comparison of Nietzsche and Plato, where Plato's imagery is frequently in tension with his thought: 'It is surprising that Plato should employ metaphors drawn from the vegetable or animal realms at all, in view of the way his metaphysics privileges the heavens and the realm of the intellect over the earth and the body' (1994: 172). A somewhat related selfreferential questioning is being sought here. The projection of space into our concepts, language and categories cannot be ignored as part of this process of dissolving abstraction into the structure of thought and affecting its concrete contents.

This problem of space is one of the projection of spatial–relational experience into the concepts and categories that underpin the frameworks of key thinkers. A static lifeless spatial experience is frequently projected. Problematising space asks questions such as: Is there a prior spatial movement, discourse or interaction pertaining to life? What are the meaningful transformations of life arising from these spatial movements? Space is to be examined as a membrane of differentiation and connection, with the diametric spatial differentiating membrane as the thick partition between self and other. In this characterisation of space as a life question, this task builds on gaps not only in the works of Nietzsche, Schopenhauer and Ricoeur, but also on silent unthought implications in Dilthey and Heidegger.

The current questioning shares with Dilthey a concern with the phenomena of life, with structures of life, life as a whole and as lived experience and, significantly, with the primary vital unity of life itself. Dilthey asks the question about a life principle in relation to the other but does not develop this issue of internalisation of the other in spatial terms.[4] Dilthey's life preoccupation with history, together with lived experience, takes a temporal turn rather than being a dynamic spatial interrogation. The focus for current purposes is less on life as selfconscious knowledge than on life spaces as preconditions for framing this awareness.[5] Where space is no longer bruised and forced into the shadows to accommodate time, the key question for current purposes is as follows: *What are the spatial principles pertaining to life?*

There is not some final endpoint 'world-eye' for life being sought or advocated for, to jounce life out of dynamism, although these spatial frames may facilitate an advocating *against* certain destructive behaviours as lacking the inclusiveness and compassion of concentric spatial relations. These spaces do not foster treatment of history deterministically as the inevitable onslaught of, for example, diametric spatial relations. Facile conclusions such as a Shelleyan 'triumph of life' must be resisted, as if a static resolution is possible rather than an ongoing, perpetual dynamic interactive tension.

It is not a paradigm that rejects the potential for constructing reality in multifarious ways, through a rigid predilection for a pregiven reality as life. Moreover, while concentric and diametric spaces may be embedded in nature as a neutral bridge language between *psyche* and *physis*,[6] they are not to be reduced simply to a flawed appeal to the 'natural'; the domain of relevance for this primordial spatial discourse is prior to the nature–culture diametric mirror image opposition or any such tropes. Life is not being treated as a substance, it is not *ousia* as presence but as a *relation*, a relational space as a *directional movement* and tension; as such, its 'presence' cannot be caged, pinned down, like dead butterflies in a museum.

Whereas early Heidegger's concerns are with how human life does not transpire in time but is time itself (2009: 265), the proposed spatial-phenomenology adapts this to argue that human life does not simply transpire *in* space but *is* space itself. Time is built into this spatial life as the proposed concentric and diametric spaces are dynamic spatial *movements*.

The scope of this book cannot embrace a questioning of life as *totality*, but is rather a scrutiny on a *unifying principle within life*, on a life movement and transformative space that engages with issues of unity and division. While others tend to treat a quest for life as unity as equivalent to a search for beauty in life (Schiller 1795; Ivanov in West 1970), so that aesthetics and life are intertwined in the fashion also of Nietzsche's goals for BT, no such assumption of an affinity between life and beauty in the search for life as unity is being held here. However, there is at least a question and hope being offered that concentric spatial movements as a direction of unity can affect and develop life quality for wellbeing – that concentric space and restructuring of diametric spatial systemic processes can offer promise for supporting wellbeing. Yet in doing so, it is not being suggested that concentric and diametric spatial processes and movements are merely anthropomorphic; it is *life* as unity and not simply human life that is the domain of relevance of these proposed primordial spaces.

Moving from the inert assumption structure of monism to the dancing interplay between living structures of diametric and concentric spaces of relation is a spatial discourse that seeks to reconstruct rather than simply deconstruct. Concentric and diametric spatial interplay is not a form or even a Schillerian living form. While this movement may bring Schillerian beauty as a unity, its function is that of a unifying direction and not necessarily beauty. Rather than being a form, it is a movement, a spatial-structural movement.[7] These concentric and diametric spaces are irreducible to Platonic ideal forms, as they are being interrogated as phenomenological structures, structures *of* experience *in* experience. These are proposed spaces of lived experience and potentialities for lived experience, where structure and content are in interplay rather than spliced into totally separate domains.

Space as a receptacle for experience awakens and enlarges the scope for experience. This paving the way for concentric space as a life-giving principle is not simply to blindly assert that the concentric can be equated with the good, Platonic or otherwise. The supposed 'goodness' or otherwise of concentric structured experience is a contextual and perspectival issue. There may be contexts where a concentric mode of experience may be too accelerated for experience or too open for interpersonal relations. Proposed as a primordial experience, it is in some way an excess on the familiar and habitual; it constitutes a struggle that brings change and this may bring its own difficulties, as part of an overall life-giving process of transformation.

Nietzsche, at least in his later work, tends to reject concepts of truth that invoke a veil to a beyond, as being metaphysical. Yet proposing diametric space as a veil for concentric space is less a veil to an abstract beyond, as *a veil to a different kind of embedded space*. It is to activate a plurality of spaces, not a monolithic spatial structure of diametric space. These spaces are not ones of sheer abstraction but are being proposed as offering an embedded immanence in shaping and constituting experience, including modes of rapturous experience.

The proposed spatial phenomenological approach seeks to expand on implications of basic foundations of Schopenhauer, Nietzsche and Ricoeur's thought. These implications are not necessarily intended by them, but are unthought latent potentialities in their work, potentialities for excavation that build on their texts rather than vaporising or dismissing their texts. Yet the goals of this process are not to recreate Schopenhauer, Nietzsche or Ricoeur's thought, but to develop a distinct vision in terms of a spatial-phenomenology building on reserves in their texts that are ripe for amplification.

There are different levels of description for concentric relational space as a systemic process of inclusion. These include intrapsychic, interpersonal and wider social systems, as well as those systems beyond direct human subjectivity, at an ontological level and in the wider physical world. To delimit the scope of the life domain being interrogated in relation to these proposed primordial spaces, it is necessary to clarify what is *not* being examined or treated as life. Concentric space is *not* being postulated as an ancient primordial experience to be re-enacted.[8] Concentric space is not as a nostalgia for the premodern or for some period of history lost in the mists of time; it is a current, ongoing experiential possibility. Life is neither being interrogated here in terms of Wittgensteinian socially constructed 'forms of life' nor Herder's nativist extolling of local cultural forms of life.

Recognising the importance of Schopenhauer's *principium individuationis*, as well as his understanding of compassion, invites challenge to Russell's dismissive account of Schopenhauer, where he treats only two features of his thought as 'historically … important' (1946: 727), Schopenhauer's pessimism and doctrine that the will is superior to knowledge.[9]

Whereas Land emphasises that Nietzsche took from Schopenhauer key insights regarding 'the elementary tenets of libidinal materialism or the philosophy of the energetic unconscious' (1991: 248), as well as the primacy of the body, aestheticism, antihumanism, misogyny, *inter alia*, the affinity between Schopenhauer and Nietzsche is being observed as significant for other particular dimensions. These are where Nietzsche engages with two core insights of Schopenhauer regarding compassion and the *principium individuationis*. Whereas the first insight regarding compassion as a connective relation to the other is thwarted by Nietzsche, the second regarding the *principium individuationis* is extolled by Nietzsche in a fashion that stretches the fabric of the Dionysian beyond previous historical manifestations. Here Nietzsche's response to key pillars of Schopenhauer's thought is one of a diametric mirror image reversal, to annihilate compassion, while accentuating the *principium individuationis*. Yet these both rest against the backdrop of Nietzsche's pervasive engagement with a third foundational pillar of Schopenhauer's thought, the will to life. Again, Nietzsche immerses himself in Schopenhauer's thought in a diametric spatial fashion, he invokes and appeals to a will to life and then arguably subsequently reverses this will to life in its service to the will to power.[10]

An ideal as concentric space is not being sought, trapped within an ideal–real opposition of abstraction; the proposed primordial spaces pertaining to life are not mere categories, static forms, collections of sterile classifications, schemes or cognitions corresponding to particular ideas, life goals or world views. Rather they are proposed as being prior framing conditions for understanding as projections of primordial experience structured through these spaces – and as such these spaces are not monoperspectival exhortations, but rather conditions for a vast plurality of perspectives to grow and thrive.

A task of this book can be conceived as one that *is paving the way for a question of wellbeing* for all people as associated with engagement in concentric spatial structures of experience and wider systems – it facilitates the question of wellbeing as concentric space, as a bounded 'freedom for' in experience, human relations, systems and life, including life systems. The issue of wellbeing, as a question of being, is one that derives from the problem of space in our structures of experience, as a dimension of a life principle through space; it prepares the ground for concentric space as a life principle of inclusion to be uncovered in human experience and existence. More precisely, it opens the way for concentric space as a life-*giving* principle as part of human existence that contains other spaces that are not life, or life-giving or supportive of life – spaces destructive of living systems, although still systems of relation themselves impinging on life systems.

Chapter 2 sets out the framework of entailments of the relative differences between concentric and diametric spaces (connection–separation, symmetry and relative openness–closure), expanding on the initial contrasts identified by Lévi-Strauss and extending these to wider domains than myths, physical and social structures. In doing so, it develops these spaces in relation to lived experience as part of a spatial-phenomenological understanding. Chapter 3 argues that a spatial-relational framework of concentric and diametric space can support Schopenhauer's compassion and defend it against the charges of egoism. A distinction between concentric spatial projections as assumed connection and diametric opposition as the 'thick partition' of assumed separation offers contrasting frames for understanding a relational self, in Schopenhauer's *Mitleid*. This challenges Nietzsche's critique of Schopenhauer's compassion as Nietzsche being locked into a diametric spatial understanding.

Dionysian rapture can be interpreted as both a collective ritual and a structure of individual experience. Early Nietzsche seeks a universal language (of music) prior to language and sets out counterpoles (Dionysian and Apollonian) in terms of relative differences as part of a complementary interplay. This invites strong parallels with differences between concentric and diametric spaces explored in Chapter 4. The question arises in this chapter as to whether this experiential shift as opening in rapture can be interpreted in terms of an interplay between diametric and concentric spaces, specifically regarding contrasts between the relative closure divorcing from interaction with background in diametric spatial systems compared with the relative openness assuming connection to background environment in concentric spatial systems. The question is interrogated in Chapter 5 as to whether Nietzsche can sustain a concentric spatial discourse of inclusion, with regard to the background *interaction* between the Dionysian and Apollonian. These background relations are argued to be understood in primordial spatial terms as the following: figure–ground as a variant of diametric space, monism, diametric spatial opposition *simpliciter*, concentric space and the void. It is proposed that these spatial dimensions are prior to Nietzsche's Dionysian–Apollonian contrasts, as a more fundamental life principle.

Chapter 6 argues that Nietzsche repeatedly illustrates the operation of will to power in spatial-structural terms as diametric space, with regard to a) diametric spatial features of splitting, and most prominently b) mirror image reversal including inversions as power hierarchy and c) closure including repetitive rituals, seeped also into the Dionysian myth in ancient Greece. Nietzsche diverts and displaces one set of diametric oppositions – good–evil – into another network of diametric spatial relations – master–slave morality, noble–base. The umbrella term of the Dionysian is used by Nietzsche to conflate the rapture of music in BT with the different rapture of the sacrificial ritual, with its killings and dances as will to power. The apparent threads of commonality between these forms of rapture as a life principle need to be unravelled through dismantling their unity in the Dionysian construct, building on Nietzsche's own disdain for forced unities.

Nietzsche's transvaluation of values challenging the traditional Platonic good, leading to free spirits beyond good and evil is examined in Chapter 7. While Nietzsche is launching an assault on habits as values, it needs to be foregrounded that he is also seeking to uproot *habits of emotion and experience.* However, he does not address here the *diametric spatial habit* that is seated throughout his accounts of fundamental experience and thought. Nietzsche's sought for experiential shift in selfovercoming is one beset by diametric space, in diametric spatial terms for experience rather than wider concentric experiential modes of transformation. Selfovercoming is a variant of the experiential restructuring already sought in overcoming the *principium individuationis* of *BT.* It is argued that whereas the experiential restructuring in the loosening from the boundaried Apollonian mode was an opening to a relation ultimately of monism with the background stormy sea of stimuli, as an annihilation of self – and a challenge to the more diametric boundaried state of the Apollonian – the later Nietzschean attempt to restructure experience operates firmly *within* a diametric spatial mode, a mirror image hierarchy.

Chapter 8 argues that the movements of concentric space are pivotal to eternal recurrence. This spatial structure emerges both at the levels of Nietzsche's imagery and concepts regarding eternal recurrence. The question is examined as to how concentric spatial movements can be related to Nietzsche's will to power as diametric spatial projections and to the Dionysian as exemplification of diametric spatial structural movements. Eternal recurrence offers a challenge to a flattened, homogenous time. This challenge commingles Nietzschean concerns with those of Charles Taylor in *A secular age*, while Taylor's preoccupation with loss of carnival as draining Western society of a life principle, offers a further resonance with Nietzsche's Dionysian thematic. These homogenous time concerns require reorientation to question homogenous space.

Chapter 9 highlights how spatial understandings pervade much of Ricoeur's discussion of living metaphor in *La Métaphore Vive*, in terms of proximity and distance, tension, substitution, displacement, change of location, image, the 'open' structure of words, closure, transparency and opaqueness. Yet this is usually where space is discussed within metaphor, and as a metaphor itself, rather than as a precondition, as a protolanguage, as prior system of relations to language interacting with language. Diametric and concentric spaces are argued to be such a prior system of relations to language, actively framing metaphor.

Chapter 10 explores conceptions of life in Ricoeur's *Oneself as another*, whether life as power, living well and with others, as well as Ricoeur's concept of embodied subjectivity as flesh that is presumably living flesh, not dead flesh. A further and arguably primordial life principle needs emphasis, namely *living space*. Ricoeur's recognition of the vital significance of space primordially, as a pivotal dimension that is even *prior* to language offers a significant conceptual leap in Ricoeur's later work. Ricoeur's proposed ontology of the flesh is one dimension towards expression of an authentic phenomenology of spatiality, albeit not necessarily the only one. Concentric and diametric spatial interplay is explored with regard to early Heidegger's existential spatiality, *Angst* and care, as candidate living spatial movements. This proposed primordial spatial discourse re-examines Ricoeur's *conatus* as power to act and his quest for a structure of relation to the other that is not closure, separation or diametric opposition, as part of an interrogation of inclusion of the other.

Notes

1 This proposed spatial protolanguage is not an attempt to rehabilitate Leibniz's claim for a protolanguage as exhibiting *ratio*, as a version of universal reason. A language of thought as such is not being sought. Leibniz sought a universal pictographic or ideographic (pictorial, diagrammatic) alphabet of human thought, complemented by calculus ratiocinator and reflecting ratio embedded in nature. In 1666 Leibniz published the dissertation *De arte combinatoria*. He wrote that all concepts (even compound ones) are only combinations of simple concepts. These concepts (just as words are compounded from letters) are extremely differentiated combinations. Leibniz considered that a language founded on the 'alphabet of human thoughts' would be possible to conduct a process of understanding using a kind of calculus, in exactly the same way as problems are solved in arithmetic or geometry. He also sought a calculating machine (*calculus ratiocinator*) that would be a tool for creating an encyclopedia of all human knowledge.

2 Regarding 'On truth and lie in an extra-moral sense' (Summer 1873), Heidegger criticises Nietzsche's influence by Schopenhauer with regard to space: 'Nietzsche, still perfectly in tune with Schopenhauer, writes that we produce representations of space and time "in us and out of us with the necessity of a spider spinning its web" (X, 202). Time too is represented subjectively and is even defined "as a property of space" (WM, 862)' (Vol. II: 90).

3 It does not avoid and evade reification, recognising the *reus* of diametric space itself as a dividing membrane into objectness (see Chapter 2). Rather, it encompasses reification to integrate the process of reification into its process of understanding, as a product of diametric spatial movement.

4 Ricoeur's questioning of a phenomenological and ontological structure of otherness offers strong resonance with a question of life in relation to the other, perhaps best expressed through Heidegger's words on Dilthey: 'Inasmuch as life is life with others, the structures of this life with one another still have to be produced. But how is this life of the other originally given?' (2009: 254), a question that Heidegger declares Dilthey never pursued further.

5 The issue of concentric and diametric space as a primordial discourse seeped into the unthought foundations of Heidegger's *Being and time*, regarding core concepts of Heidegger in this work, including encountering and side by sideness, authenticity and inauthenticity; *Angst*, care, the transcendental horizon of temporality, have been interrogated elsewhere (Downes 2012).
6 As sought by Nobel prize-winning physicist, Wolfgang Pauli, see Downes (2016) for a preliminary exploration of these spaces in biology and quantum physics, as well as Downes (2006, 2010, 2012) on Newtonian physics and diametric space.
7 Whereas form divides from content, structure in concentric space is continuous with content in a radical fashion so that what is perceived as structure and what as content depends on the relativity of the vantage point in an expanding network of structure–content relations (see Lévi-Strauss 1963; Downes 2010, 2012 on structure–content relativity).
8 See also Downes (2012) on a range of different meanings to the term primordial.
9 Somewhat in contrast to Russell, Kaufmann not only views sublimation as of 'central significance' for Nietzsche's later philosophy, including for selfovercoming as the problem of overcoming the impulses, Kaufmann acknowledges Schopenhauer's antecedent insight and potential influence in Schopenhauer's reference to 'representations' 'sublimated into abstract concepts' (1975: 219).
10 Copleston describes much of the relation between Schopenhauer and Nietzsche in terms that are tantamount to a diametric mirror image inverted relation: 'That there is a gulf between Schopenhauer and Nietzsche is undeniable, for the one preaches resignation, the other defiance, the one conformity, denial, asceticism, the other rebellion, affirmation, strength and action' (1942/1975: 158).

References

Copleston, F., *Friedrich Nietzsche: Philosopher of Culture*. New York: Barnes & Noble Books, 1942/1975.

de Beauvoir, S., *The Second Sex*. New York: Vintage, 1949/1989.

Descartes, R., *Descartes: Philosophical Writings*. Trans. E. Anscombe and P. T. Geach. London: Nelson, 1954.

Downes, P., 'Newtonian Space: The "Blind Spot" in Newell and Simon's Information Processing Paradigm', *Cybernetics and Human Knowing*, 2006,13: 25–55.

Downes, P., 'Schema Structure–Content Relativity: Part II, From Image Schemata to Background Spatial Schemata of Diametric and Concentric Relation', *Cybernetics and Human Knowing*, 2010,17: 25–43.

Downes, P., *The Primordial Dance: Diametric and Concentric Spaces in the Unconscious World*. Oxford/Bern: Peter Lang, 2012.

Downes, P., 'Concentric and Diametric Spatial Structures of Relation: Exploring a Neutral Bridge Language between Quantum Physics and Neuropsychology', *Neuroquantology, An Interdisciplinary Journal of Neuroscience and Quantum Physics*, 2016, 14(3).

Fitch, W. T., *The Evolution of Language*. Cambridge: Cambridge University Press, 2010.

Heidegger, M., *Nietzsche*, Vols I and II. D. F. Krell (ed.), trans. D. F. Krell. New York: HarperCollins, 1991.

Heidegger, M., 'Wilhelm Dilthey's Research and the Current Struggle for a World-view', in T. Kisiel and T. Sheehan (eds.), *Becoming Heidegger: On the Trail of His Early Occasional Writings 1910–1927*. Seattle: Noesis Press, 2nd revised, expanded ed., 2009.

Kaufmann, W., *Nietzsche: Philosopher, Psychologist, Antichrist.* Princeton, NJ: Princeton University Press, 4th ed., 1975.

Kearney, R., 'Paul Ricoeur and the Hermeneutics of Translation', *Research in Phenomenology*, 2007,37: 147–159.

Körner, S., 'The Impossibility of Transcendental Deductions', *Monist,* 1967,51: 317–331.

Land, N., 'Art as Insurrection: The Question of Aesthetics in Kant, Schopenhauer and Nietzsche', in K. Ansell-Pearson (ed.), *Nietzsche and Modern German Thought.* London: Routledge, 1991, 240–256.

Lévi-Strauss, C., *The Savage Mind*, trans. G. Weidenfeld, Nicolson Ltd. Chicago, IL: Chicago University Press, 1962.

Lévi-Strauss, C., *Structural Anthropology*, Vol. 1., trans. C. Jacobsen and B. Grundfest Schoepf. London: Penguin. 1963.

Lévi-Strauss, C., *Structural Anthropology*, Vol. 2., trans. M. Layton. London: Penguin Books, 1973.

Parkes, G., *Composing the Soul: Reaches of Nietzsche's Psychology*. Chicago, IL: University of Chicago Press, 1994.

Pauli, W., *Atom and Archetype: The Pauli-Jung Letters 1932–1958.* C. A. Meier (ed.), trans. D. Roscoe. London: Routledge, 2001.

Russell, B., *A History of Western Philosophy and its Connection with Political and Social Circumstances from the Earliest Times to the Present Day*. London: George Allen & Unwin, 1946/1983.

Said, E. W., *Orientalism*. London: Routledge & Kegan Paul, 1978.

Schiller, F., *On the Aesthetic Education of Man. tr.* E. M.Wilkinson and L.A. Willoughby *(eds.), trans.* E. M.Wilkinson and L. A. Willoughby. Oxford: Clarendon Press, 1795/1982.

West, J., *Russian Symbolism: A Study of Vyacheslav Ivanov and the Russian Symbolist Aesthetic*. London: Methuen, 1970.

Chapter 2

Features of the spatial protolanguage of concentric and diametric space

Concentric and diametric space as a protolanguage of relation: beyond space as a shadow text

Early Nietzsche seeks to extract structural contrasts as part of two myths, the Dionysian and Apollonian. The structural contrasts embedded in these myths are purportedly a prior fundamental 'eternal' discourse, at least for tragedy and for aesthetic purposes viewed 'through the optic of life' (BT: 5). Such an approach of search for prior structural contrasts between myths was taken up by Lévi-Strauss, without invoking any debt to Nietzsche, explicitly or implicitly, and accelerated into a focus on contrasts across wider cross-cultural myths and mythic contrasts. Without needing to take on board the epistemological commitments of Lévi-Strauss' structuralist reliance on linguistics for interpreting myths, or all of his accounts of such contrasts, it is Lévi-Strauss' key explications of diametric and concentric structures of relation in myth, as well as in physical structures, across diverse cultures that open up a new horizon of questioning pertaining to a protolanguage of space. Lévi-Strauss apprehended this spatial horizon in rudimentary fashion, without addressing its potential ramifications for a wider ambit of relevance.

Lévi-Strauss tended to discuss concentric and diametric structures as structures and not so much as *spaces*. Developing an aspect of Lévi-Strauss' (1962, 1963, 1973) understanding of structures of relation (Downes 2012, 2013), space is to be examined as an interactive tension between diametric and concentric spaces of relation. A diametric spatial structure is one where a circle is split in half by a line that is its diameter or where a square or rectangle is similarly divided into two equal halves (see Figure 2.1). In a concentric spatial structure, one circle is inscribed in another larger circle (or square); in pure form, the circles share a common central point (see Figure 2.2).

A purportedly key distinguishing feature of concentric and diametric structures, observed by Lévi-Strauss, is that they tend to coexist in 'functional relation' (1973: 73) and not simply in isolation. They are structures of relation as part of a system of relations. Being mutually interactive, at least potentially, they are observed as structures *of* relation but also structures *in* relation. Lévi-

Figure 2.1 Diametric dualism

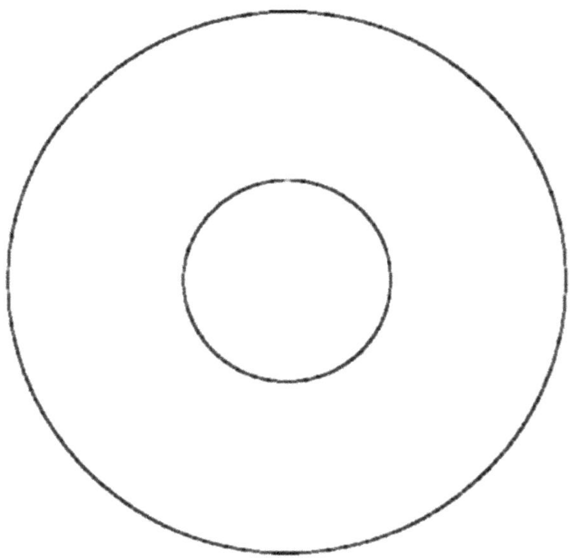

Figure 2.2 Concentric dualism

Strauss recognises that they are fundamentally interlinked, so that an increase in one is compensated for by decrease in the other. Meaning is in their contrasting relative differences, rather than in either space considered in isolated, absolute, atomistic or essentialist terms. Lévi-Strauss opened up a discourse of relation between concentric and diametric structures, without apprehending the potentially wider scope of this spatial discourse, as it becomes transferred to other contexts of relation.

Ricoeur comments on French structuralism in general, contrasting it with Husserlian phenomenology:

> [T]he *linguistic turn* … has often signified a refusal to 'go outside' of language and a mistrust equal to that of French structuralism with respect to any extralinguistic order … the implicit axiom that everything is language has often led to a closed semanticism, incapable of accounting for human action as actually happening in the world … a phenomenology like Husserl's, according to which the stratum of language is ineffectual in relation to the life of intentional consciousness, has a corrective value, just because it proposes the opposite extreme. (OA: 301)

Ricoeur signals some distance from the linguistic turn. He displays on openness to a level prior to or, at least, beyond language, while situating French structuralism and hence Lévi-Strauss, as locked within linguistic assumptions, although overlooking that his concentric and diametric structural relations were in some way prior to language; this feature of concentric and diametric relations being prior to language was, however, not emphasised by Lévi-Strauss. It would seem that Lévi-Strauss overlooked concentric and diametric structures as a discourse fundamentally of space due to his own structuralist commitments to the primacy of language.

Resonant with the Janus face of two heads looking in diametrically opposite directions in Greek mythology, Lévi-Strauss notes that examples of diametric dualism 'abound' (1962: 135), citing specific tribes in North and South America. Moreover, the simple everyday cross-cultural oppositions between 'good' and 'bad' are structured in a diametric oppositional way. The diametric good–bad opposition also underlies myths such as those of the Shuswap, which treats the owl as a cannibalistic monster in contrast to the Kutenai, which treats the owl as a benefactor (Lévi-Strauss 1973). Lévi-Strauss (1963) cites a range of examples of the concentric spatial opposition observed by different anthropologists. These include: the village plan of Omarakana in the Trobriand Islands, published by Malinowski; the Baduj of western Java and the Negri-Sembilan of the Malay peninsula, observed by de Jong; the village of the Winnebago tribe observed by Radin and an archaeological finding in the Lower Mississippi Valley.

Concentric structures can be found also in Islamic, Japanese, Russian, Chinese, Jewish, Celtic, African, ancient Greek and Estonian contexts (Downes 2003, 2012), while Jung (1936/1985) locates the concentric mandala structure in Buddhist, Hindu and Christian traditions. With regard to the Lower Mississippi Valley, Lévi-Strauss states:

> We are therefore dealing with a type of [concentric] structure which in America extends far back into antiquity, and whose later analogues were to be found in preConquest Peru and Bolivia and … in the social structure of the Sioux in North America and of the Ge and related tribes in South America. (1963: 143)

This latter structure, however, was not simply bipolar but 'forming six concentric octagonal figures' (Lévi-Strauss 1963: 143). Myriad cross-cultural examples of concentric space as an ancient structure embedded in human experience can be found.

Diametric and concentric projected spatial structures of relation: assumed separation and assumed connection

A claim is not being made that the entailments of the relational differences between concentric and diametric spaces are qualities that are in some way essential or intrinsic to either structure, considered as individual isolated structures, abstracted from the context of their mutual relation. A key relative difference, overlooked by Lévi-Strauss' empiricism, is nevertheless, ascertainable in principle. It is evident that the inner and outer poles of concentric space are fundamentally attached to one another, unlike in diametric space. It is a self-evident entailment of concentric relation that both concentric poles coexist in the same space, and thus, the outer circle overlaps the space of the inner one; the outer circle surrounds and contains the inner circle. The opposite that is within the outer circle or shape cannot detach itself from being within this outer shape. That the outer circle or shape can move in the direction of greater detachment from the inner circle notwithstanding, it cannot, in principle, fully detach itself from the inner circle in concentric relation (even if the inner circle becomes an increasingly smaller proportion of the outer). Full detachment could conceivably occur only through destroying or altering the form of the other pole. It can be concluded that full detachment could occur only through destroying the very concentric structure of the whole opposition itself.

In contradistinction, in diametric space both oppositional realms are basically detached and can be further smoothly detached from the other. These conclusions operate for both spaces, whether they are viewed as being two dimensional or three dimensional. A concentric space assumes connection between its parts and any separation is on the basis of assumed connection, whereas diametric space assumes separation and any connection between the parts is on the basis of this assumed separation. As structures in relational difference, this contrast is a relativistic one of degree (Downes 2012, 2013). Concentric and diametric spaces thus can be seen to offer contrasting structures of differential relation. A concentric spatial relation is a structure of inclusion compared to a diametric spatial structure of exclusion. In Bachelard's words, pertinent to diametric space, 'simple geometrical opposition becomes tinged with aggressivity' (1964: 212). This is not a predilection for geometrical or mathematical models in general, rather, it is for this specific spatial system of relations based on geometric contrasts meaningful also for experience.

Interpreting these spatial structures dynamically as movements, as *spatial movements*, brings an implication of diametric space as assumed separation, namely, that it involves a movement of splitting, of imposing relations of splitting as part of the assumed separation built into its structure. Diametric space, in contrast to concentric space, brings a change to a system in the direction of fostering a splitting process, rather than developing a relational movement of assumed connection as that of a concentric spatial system. These spaces are being examined as fundamentally directions of movement rather than to be treated as simply static structures.

A Japanese cultural context illustrates the entwinement between the spatial and the relational. Morioka suggests that 'the idea of inside/outside is not only a radical essential category of cultural characteristics, but [is] also universal' (2007: 193), citing Kimura's (2005) emphasis that the Japanese words *uchi* (inside) and *soto* (outside) express a characteristic cultural ethos, where *uchi* (inside) is exactly equal to that of one's family or group. Yet a diametric outsideness is an assumed separation that is radically different from the assumed connection of the outside pole to the inner pole of concentric space. Inner and outer need not necessarily be diametrically framed but may also be concentrically framed. The Japanese concept of *ma* can signify the space between one thing and another and can also be used for an understanding of human relationships (Morioka 2007). Concentric and diametric spatial structures of relation invite application to relations between self and other, thereby entwining the spatial and relational, as with the Japanese concept *ma*.

To oppose is a position in space, the op-positional space of diametricity. Thomson summarizes Heidegger's insight into this assumed separation: 'As Heidegger frequently points out, in the modern, post-Cartesian world, an "object", *Gegenstand*, is something that "stands opposite" a human subject, something *external* to subjectivity' (2011: 49). Diametric spatial relation is such a standing opposite; the diametric poles are juxtaposed, opposite one another. Perhaps influenced by Heidegger, Fromm makes a related point: 'I – the observer – stand against my "ob-ject" … in German, *Gegenstand* = "counter-stand"' (1962: 149). Diametric poles exemplify such ob-jectification and reification as they counterstand against one another in opposition; a spatial precondition for objectification is diametric space.

The assumed separation of diametric space must be distinguished from the nonrelation of discordance, highlighted by Heidegger in his readings of Nietzsche: 'Only two things that are related to one other can be opposed to each other. But such opposition is not yet discordance' (Vol. I: 189). Heidegger continues that 'severance is something different from opposition' (Vol. I: 189). Diametric space is still a relation of a kind, even in its mode of splitting as a dynamic process of assumed separation. Splitting assumes either a prior connection or at least the potential for a connection. In contrast, as Heidegger highlights there are modes of discordance in which no relation as such is possible, adopting spatial imagery to describe discordance in terms of a 'gap' 'split' 'cliffs' (Vol. I: 189); even the capacity for opposition cannot exist as there is no supporting condition of diametric space.

These ancient concentric and diametric structures of relation in relation share with language the feature of being a transsubjective system of relations. However, as a discourse of implication, this does not make the spatial dualisms reducible to a linguistic system. The examination of them here is to develop a position beyond Lévi-Strauss' structuralism, rather than simply echoing his fundamental assumptions. For example, the relational difference between the assumed connection of concentric space and the assumed separation of diametric oppositional space need not be subsumed by the Procrustean force of a claimed commitment of Lévi-Strauss to Cartesian mental structures, noted by D'Aquili (1975). It may have been these very commitments to rigid Cartesian dichotomies that led to Lévi-Strauss overlooking the key entailment that concentric relation challenges such dichotomies and is more connective than diametric relation.

It is important to emphasise that Lévi-Strauss' account of diverse empirical observations of concentric and diametric spatial structures is but one small part of his structural anthropological project and it is to be recognised that his project is open to a number of criticisms (Derrida 1974, 1978); the argument being developed is not one that requires commitment to accepting other aspects of Lévi-Strauss' work such as ahistorical truth claims (see Downes 2012, 2013 on how concentric and diametric spaces can avoid Derrida's general criticisms of Lévi-Strauss' structuralist assumptions). It was in Lévi-Strauss' cross-cultural accounts of *systems*, whether physical, social structures or mythological, where dynamic relations of contrast between concentric and diametric structures of relation began to be made more explicit. However, Lévi-Strauss did not realise the full potential of his systemic insights or interrogate the transferability of these dynamic diametric and concentric spaces to other kinds of system of relation. He tended to treat diametric and concentric modes as structures and underemphasised their features as spaces and as dynamic spatial systems.

Diametric space as mirror image inversion and its relation with concentric space

Lévi-Strauss describes 'symmetrical inversions' (1973: 247) in Mandan and Hidatsa myths:

> [...] these myths are diametrically opposed ... In the Mandan version ... two earth women who are not sisters go to heaven to become sisters-in-law by marrying celestial brothers. One who belongs to the Mandan tribe, separates from an ogre, Sun, with the help of a string which enables her to come back down to her village. In revenge, Sun places his legitimate son at the head of the enemies of the Mandan, upon whom he declares war. In the Hidatsa version ... everything is exactly reversed. Two celestial brothers come down to earth to be conceived by human beings and born

> as children. Sun's sister, an ogress, is joined with an earthborn character by means of a string. She makes him her adopted son and puts him at the head of the enemies of the Hidatsa. (1973: 250)

He reiterates a view of diametric structural opposition as expressing qualities of inverted symmetry, when contrasting the myth of the Thompson and the Coeur d'Alene with that of the Chilcotin (1973: 262). Echoing a view of symmetry as 'transformations which sometimes result in the meaning being turned inside out', he invokes descriptions of myths, framed by an understanding of their relation as involving, what amounts to a mirror image:

> One often observes ... that mythological systems after passing through a minimal expression, recover their original fullness on the other side of the threshold. But their reflection is inverted a bit like a bundle of light rays entering into a camera obscura through a pin-point opening and forced by this obstacle to cross over each other. The same image seen rightside-up outside is reflected upside-down in the camera. (Lévi-Strauss 1973: 259–260)

A mirror image is not an identical one but a left–right inversion. Strictly speaking, a mirror image is plane symmetry, rather than the line symmetry of diametric dualism. Nevertheless, plane, line and point symmetry all accommodate a view of symmetry as reversal or inversion. While Lévi-Strauss (1970: 31) acknowledges the need for greater precision within his use of terms such as symmetry, it was a key concept in much of his work (1963, 1970, 1973). While Lévi-Strauss related diametric structured, mirror image symmetry to myths, concentric spatial structures of relation are not a symmetry as inversion. Rather, they offer a different entailment of symmetry as unity, where the line or axis of symmetry brings the same pole rather than a mirror image pole in diametric structures.

Music is treated by Nietzsche as 'a universal language' (BT: 87), with 'music the power to give birth once again to myth' (BT: 93). It is evident that myth is not a universal language for Nietzsche;[1] he treats music as a universal language prior to myth and to language, concept and representation. Similarly, Lévi-Strauss' concentric and diametric spaces unfold a pattern in myth that is prior to myth, as being more fundamental than myth itself.

It is notable that at the very outset of Volume II of WWR, Schopenhauer's first sentence conceives of the world in concentric structured terms: 'In endless spaces countless luminous spheres, round each of which some dozen smaller illuminated ones revolve ... those numberless spheres' (WWRII: 3). Strikingly a fundamental conclusion of this volume is made in diametric mirror image oppositional terms, somewhat resonant with Kantian antinomies:

> What gives life its strange and ambiguous character is that in it two fundamental purposes, diametrically opposed, are constantly crossing each other. One purpose is that of the individual will, directed to chimerical happiness in an ephemeral, dreamlike, and deceptive existence ... The other purpose is that of fate, directed obviously enough to the destruction of our happiness, and thus to the mortification of our will, and to the elimination of the delusion that holds us chained to the bonds of this world. (WWRII: 638–639)

While framing conditions for understanding, these concentric and diametric spaces do not themselves constitute a distinctive worldview, set of life goals or thoughts as cognitions. They are precognitive framing spaces and are prior to metaphor.[2]

Parkes (1994) highlights Nietzsche's words from the opening page of the essay *On the Use and Disadvantage of History for Life: Untimely Meditations* 2, on 'the horizon that every living being has to draw around itself in order to survive' and develops this point: 'There is a need for a kind of membrane to separate self from other, inner from outer, the present moment from the past and future; and the health of the living being will depend on the permeability of that membrane and its flexibility with respect to expansions and contractions' (1994: 102). Building on Nietzsche's conception of the horizon, Parkes relates this membrane not only to issues of separation but also permeability and expansion. This offers a strong resonance with another feature of diametric and concentric space highlighted by Lévi-Strauss with regard to closure and openness in interaction with background.

Third entailment of the relative differences between concentric and diametric spaces: foreground–background interaction versus noninteraction

Another feature of diametricity, contrasted with concentric space, is highlighted by Lévi-Strauss. He argues that self-sufficiency and a split relation to the outside environment is a general quality of diametric structures and systems: 'In a diametric system ... virgin land constitutes an irrelevant element; the moieties are defined by their opposition to each other, and the apparent symmetry of their closed structure creates the illusion of a closed system' (Lévi-Strauss 1963: 152). While this makes sense for the immediate example given for social structures, it is not yet clear if non-self-sufficiency and orientation to the outside environment is a general quality of concentric as opposed to diametric relation, as Lévi-Strauss claims:

> [In concentric relation] the system is not self-sufficient, and its frame of reference is always the environment. The opposition between cleared ground (central circle) and waste land (peripheral circle) demands a third

> element, brush or forest – that is, virgin land – which circumscribes the binary whole while at the same time extending it, since cleared land is to waste land as waste land is to virgin land. (1963: 152)

Lévi-Strauss rejects closure for concentric structures, by implying that the relation of the background to both poles of the dualism is governed by the relation within the dualism itself, i.e., 'cleared land is to waste land as waste land is to [background] virgin land'. The mode of relation to the background is not extraneous to the respective modes of relation within the poles themselves. Thus, as the concentric poles are in assumed connection to each other, they are also in assumed connection to the background; and this assumed connection to the background resists closure within the concentric structure. In contrast, diametric structures' relation to their own poles is one of assumed separation that then maintains an assumed separation with the background.

There is minimal interaction between the structural poles of diametric relation and the background space (i.e., virgin land). Diametric structures' relation to their own poles is one of a mirror image division, which then maintains a cleavage from the background that becomes closed off. Moreover, diametric and concentric structures are dynamic processes as much as structures. Thus, a diametric structure tends to impose a diametric process in its interaction with the background, whereas a concentric structure initiates a concentric relation with the background. In this sense of involvement with the background, concentric relation is not a self-contained structure. There is a closer proximity between background and foreground within concentric relative to diametric space. In comparison, diametric space is a much more closed structure – closed off from the background. There is greater closure in a diametric spatial structure relative to a dis-closure process of relative opening in concentric spatial relation. A variant of the entailment of relative closure for diametric structures is that they bring decreased permeability (transparency) relative to the increased permeability (transparency) of concentric structures. The more fluid open boundaries of concentric space are more permeable and transparent than the hard-walled boundaries of diametric space.

The proposed primordial spatial discourse of concentric and diametric structured relations underpinning experience is being postulated as a fundamental universal protolanguage. Very basic aspects of experience (connection–separation, symmetry, relative openness–closure) are meaningful in spatial terms and cluster into a protolanguage of concentric and diametric spaces as differential contrasts. Entailments of the differences between concentric and diametric spaces (connection–separation, symmetry, relative openness–closure) are being proposed as elemental features as conditions of experience. Another dimension of foreground–background interaction with regard to diametric spatial closure and concentric spatial openness, recognised in Downes (2012) is with regard to such closure and openness as pertaining to permeability and transparency.

Gestalt figure–ground spatial relations as a variant of diametric space

The well-known artistic distinction between figure and ground is illustrated in the ambiguous figure (Figure 2.3) devised by the Danish psychologist Edgar Rubin.

Hofstadter's discussion of the figure–ground distinction highlights the importance of foreground–background interaction for Gestalt psychology:

> When a figure or positive space (e.g., a human form, or a letter, or a still life) is drawn inside a frame, an unavoidable consequence is that its complementary shape also called the 'ground' or 'background' or 'negative space' has also been drawn. In most drawings, however, the figure–ground relationship plays little role. The artist is much less interested in the ground than the figure. But sometimes, an artist will take interest in the ground as well. (1979: 67)

Hofstadter states the need to distinguish between two kinds of figure: cursively drawable ones and recursive ones. A cursively drawable figure is one whose ground [space] is merely an accidental by-product of the drawing act. A recursive figure is one whose ground [space] can be seen as a figure in its own right. This tends to be quite deliberate on the part of the artist.

The question arises as to the relationship between the Gestalt figure–ground and diametric and concentric spaces. The interaction between Gestalt figure and ground is *not* one where the ground tends to *surround* the figure (e.g., face to vase, the face does not surround the vase) unlike the outer concentric structure surrounding the inner concentric structure. The realm for active interaction between Gestalt figure and ground is limited to one side only of

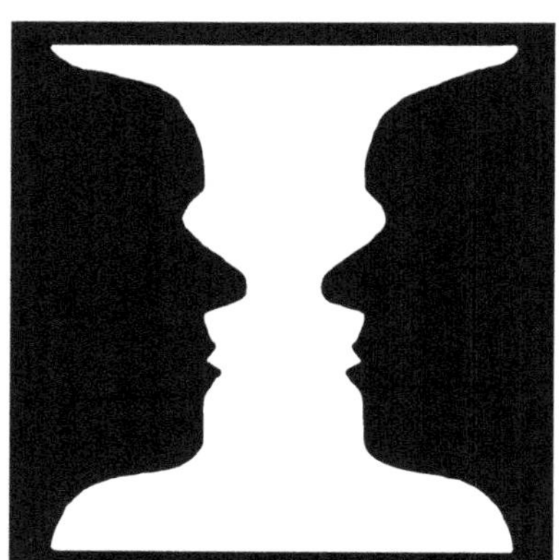

Figure 2.3 Gestalt figure–ground spatial relations

each shape – there are still two distinct halves in the Gestalt figure–ground as with diametric rather than concentric space. Moreover, these two halves can be smoothly detached from one another without losing their overall structure as with diametric space. The shape of each is only mutually self-defining in a limited sense, namely, that their interactive mutuality depends on the closure and definition of the other parts of both figure and ground – the parts that are not in active interaction. Only a limited aspect of both poles engage with the other in figure–ground interaction. This all highlights that the Gestalt figure–ground is more a diametric than concentric structure.

It is arguably, however, a less extreme form of diametric relation, as there is at least the implication of a reciprocal, complementary relation between both aspects, the figure and ground in their mutual self-defining roles. On a view of concentric relation as a trajectory for change to diametric relation, a figure–ground diametric relation illustrates a dimension of movement from diametric relation *simpliciter* in its interplay with the process of concentric relational space.

It is the mirror image part not the dualism part that is the movement, the first breath of movement. So from monism to diametric opposition is a spatial movement at least for the mirror image inversion aspect. The projection of diametric experiential space into thought is an animating movement of sorts, it is a movement as projection so it has some life aspect in this limited sense and it expresses mirror image symmetry. Is early Nietzsche's preoccupation with the primacy of the aesthetic in relation to not only tragedy but life, a displaced version of a quest for a prior truth domain of the spatial, that could be construed as a spatial aesthetic?

These spatial structures of relation are a shadow text on the text in the sense that they open a space, a dimension that is spatial within the flesh of the text, so the text is no longer flat but is a three-dimensional spatial phenomenon. A shadow requires something more than a flattened two-dimensional space. In the sense that they offer a dimensional opening, these spatial structures give flesh to the text. Yet this is not some paradox that a shadow gives flesh, a description of these background spatial structures as shadows is mere analogy. The disanalogy within the analogy must be brought to the fore. This is not a shadow text in the sense that a shadow derives from light, such as shadows on the wall of a Platonic cave. The space is not derivative (from light) as a shadow is, rather it is being postulated as a protolanguage that is prior to language – it is prior as being primordial. Primordial here is not being invoked in terms of some ancient prehistory. This spatial dimension is proposed as ontologically prior and primordial as a more fundamental truth or experience; a direction of unity for experience; a truth and experience prior to socially constructed realities; a cross-cultural truth; being beyond the limited schema of causal explanations (see also Downes 2012).

These proposed primordial spatial structures open up a vista of background–foreground interaction as an expansive dimension for understanding truth claims (where which is seen as more pivotal and which is seen as derivative depends on the vantage point of the perceiver and the truth goals of the observer). It is the background set of spaces that have been neglected and have remained largely in the shadows of Western thought, thereby constituting a fleshless, flattened Western thought.

The focus in a spatial-phenomenology is not on a 'beyond' the text but on an accelerated immanence within the text to acutely expose spatial horizons. These proposed primordial spaces do not simply invade the basic concepts of Schopenhauer, Nietzsche and Ricoeur's seminal works or merely house these basic concepts. These spaces actively constitute the basic concepts, so that structure and content are entwined, so that it is not a mere matter of form and content. Space is interactively imbued within the content, not as an addendum but in a pivotal and pervasive manner. An assumption structure for basic concepts is not mere metaphor, but can be laid bare in spatial terms. Metaphor is a mediating movement towards an opening of space into three-dimensional thought.

Concentric space, as a fragile potential, is in dynamic interactive relation with power dimensions, so it is not a case of a pre-established harmony as a jigsaw to be pieced together. Concentric and diametric space are not sheer presences, locked into a truth as *ousia* claim as a substance ontology. These spaces are not being treated as 'homes' for experience, there is no simple primordial home as such; the very mode of their interrelation implies that neither offers a presence or completeness to be a static home for experience. This spatial protolanguage offers structures of difference, of differential relation where space is the medium of difference, the medium as differential relation to hold difference in the grasp of understanding.

Notes

1 Parkes associates Nietzsche's lack of later explicit discussion of myth as part of his ultimate distancing from Wagner who extolled myth (1994: 83).

2 Nietzsche aptly recognises '*how late* are more acute logical thinking, a rigorous application of cause and effect, developed; *even now*, our functions of reason and intelligence reach back instinctively to those primitive forms of deductions' (HH: 22). For diametric space as a primordial structural precondition for cause–effect and Aristotelian A/non-A logic, see Downes (2010, 2012).

References

Bachelard, G., *The Poetics of Space*. Boston, MA: Beacon Press, 1964/1994.

D'Aquili, E., 'The Influence of Jung on the Work of Claude Lévi-Strauss', *Journal of the History of the Behavioral Sciences*, 1975, 11: 41–48.

Derrida, J., *Of Grammatology*. London/Baltimore, MA: Johns Hopkins University Press, 1974.

Derrida, J., *Writing and Difference*. Trans. A. Bass. London: Routledge & Kegan Paul, 1978/1981.

Downes, P., 'Cross-Cultural Structures of Concentric and Diametric Dualism in Lévi-Strauss' Structural Anthropology: Structures of Relation Underlying the Self and Ego Relation?', *Journal of Analytical Psychology*, 2003, 48: 47–81.

Downes, P', 'Schema Structure-Content Relativity: Part II, From Image Schemata to Background Spatial Schemata of Diametric and Concentric Relation', *Cybernetics and Human Knowing*, 2010,17: 25–43.
Downes, P., *The Primordial Dance: Diametric and Concentric Spaces in the Unconscious World*. Oxford/Bern: Peter Lang, 2012.
Downes, P., 'Developing Derrida's Psychoanalytic Graphology: Diametric and Concentric Spatial Movements', *Derrida Today*, 2013,6(2): 197–221.
Fromm, E., *Beyond the Chains of Illusion: My Encounter with Marx and Freud*. New York: Continuum, 1962/1990.
Heidegger, M., *Nietzsche*, Vols I and II. D. F. Krell (ed.), trans. D. F. Krell. New York: HarperCollins, 1991.
Hofstadter, D. R., *Godel, Escher, Bach: An Eternal Golden Braid*. New York: Basic Books, 1979.
Hofstadter, D., *Metamagical Themas: Quests for the Essence of Mind and Pattern*. New York: Basic Books, 1985.
Jung, C. G., 'Individual Dream Symbolism in Relation to Alchemy'. InC. G. Jung, *Dreams*. London: Ark, 1936/1985.
Kimura, B., *Kankei tositeno jiko* [The Self as Relationships]. Tokyo: Misuzu syobo, 2005.
Krell, D. F., 'Introduction to the Paperback Edition', in M. Heidegger, *Nietzsche*, Vols I and II. D. F. Krell (ed.), trans. D. F. Krell. New York: HarperCollins, 1991, ix–xxvii.
Lévi-Strauss, C., *The Savage Mind*. Trans. G. Weidenfeld, Nicolson Ltd. Chicago: Chicago University Press, 1962/1966.
Lévi-Strauss, C., *Structural Anthropology, Vol. 1*. Trans. C. Jacobsen and B. Grundfest Schoepf. London: Penguin, 1963.
Lévi-Strauss, C., *The Raw and the Cooked: Introduction to a Science of Mythology* I. London: Jonathan Cape, 1970.
Lévi-Strauss, C., *Structural Anthropology, Vol. 2*. Trans. M. Layton. London: Penguin, 1973/1977.
Morioka, M., 'Commentary: Constructing Creative Appropriations', *Culture & Psychology*, 2007,13: 189–196.
Parkes, G., *Composing the Soul: Reaches of Nietzsche's Psychology*. Chicago, IL: University of Chicago Press, 1994.
Thomson, I. D., *Heidegger, Art and Modernity*. New York: Cambridge University Press, 2011.

Chapter 3

Compassion and space

The reduction of Schopenhauer's distinctive concept of compassion to egoism: a debate resting on primordial spatial assumptions of concentric and diametric space

The elegance of space staggers in the shadows of a key difference between Schopenhauer and Nietzsche, where Nietzsche launches an assault on even the possibility of compassion in Schopenhaurean terms. This issue runs to the kernel of human potentialities, concerning life and inclusion.

The key dimension of compassion (*Mitleid*) in a shift from egoism is a core distinctive tenet of Schopenhauer's philosophical corpus, including *On The Basis of Morality* and the Fourth Book of Schopenhauer's main work, *The World as Will and Representation*. Schopenhauer treats compassion (*Mitleid*) and suffering as metaphysical states, which he distinguished from the psychological. It is important to emphasise, with Bobko (2001: 95), that compassion is not only central to Schopenhauer's metaphysics but also to his view of an original experience of the moral.

For Schopenhauer, each individual is an expression of will striving to fulfil its ultimate drive towards life. Schopenhauer broadly espouses much of Kant's transcendental idealism, emphasising key Kantian principles such as that ultimately, space and time are exclusively subjective forms of our *a priori* intuition; while the world of representation is individuated spatio-temporally, the world as it is in itself lies 'outside' of space and time. Building on this Kantian edifice, for Schopenhauer, the thing in itself is 'one' and is best described as 'Will'. Ultimately, we are 'one' with each other qua objectifications of Will; the person with a strong capacity for compassion intuitively understands this.

Against this backdrop, it is notable that with regard to compassion, Schopenhauer directly contradicts Kant who treats feeling of compassion as a weakness (WWRI: 402). Schopenhauer is not seeking a universal Kantian formula for duty, he explicitly rejects search for an unconditional ought for morality offering instead his pivotal notion of compassion. In doing so, he is shifting the key domain of relevance for morality away from 'abstract cognition' (WWRI: 395) and towards experience of compassion.[1] Moreover,

Schopenhauer's view of the metaphysical is a distinctive one that treats the metaphysical as being central to experience. For Schopenhauer, experience of suffering is a key to recognition of the 'world'. Schopenhauer's link between metaphysics and experience is a break with traditional conceptions of rationalistic, *a priori* metaphysics, diverging here from Kant and providing an ancestry for Husserl.

Schopenhauer's thematising of compassion describes a central feature as, 'the immediate participation ... primarily in the suffering of another' (OBM: 144/208f.). He continues:

> As soon as this compassion is aroused, the weal and woe of another are nearest to my heart in exactly the same way, although not always in exactly the same degree, as otherwise only my own are. Hence the difference between him and me is now no longer absolute. (OBM: 144/208f.)

The kernel of Schopenhauer's analysis of compassion is that a person participates immediately in another's suffering.

As Cartwright (2008) notes, a pervasive theme among critics historically, including Johann August Becker, Nietzsche and Max Scheler, is that Schopenhauer engages in an unwitting reduction of compassion to some form of egoism. In Young's words, such compassion is in the interests of his 'metaphysical rather than his empirical self' so that the person becomes a 'metaphysical egoist' (2005: 182f.). Young's framing of the question in terms of a metaphysical self already runs into a conflict with Schopenhauer, as for Schopenhauer if one means by metaphysical self, one's substance as the will that underlies everything, then there is no personality or self involved at all, since individuality is completely dissolved at the basic metaphysical level. The key aspect of Young's critique at issue here is his characterisation of compassion, echoing Nietzsche, in terms of reduction merely to egoism. This chapter will argue that the spatial-phenomenological framework of concentric space contrasted with diametric space can support Schopenhauer's conception of compassion and defend it against the charges of egoism.

Nietzsche's criticisms of Schopenhauer's *Mitleid* refer to, 'the follies of the compassionate' (Z: 114). He asks, 'Why double your "ego"! ... to view and imbibe the experiences of others as if they were ours', as is the 'demand of a philosophy' of *Mitleid*. With characteristic bombast, he concludes, 'this would destroy us' (D: §137). For current purposes, it is Nietzsche's framing of compassion as a doubling of the ego that is at issue. Challenge here to Nietzsche's view of compassion as an accentuation of the ego does not focus on other criticisms of compassion given by Nietzsche in terms of its lack of utility,[2] its expression of a slave morality viewed as pervading Judaeo-Christian traditions or how compassion may mask power relations. Some commentators have raised concerns as to whether the focus of critique of Nietzsche on Schopenhauer's *Mitleid* was on pity rather than compassion (see Janaway 2007 for an account of this issue). For current purposes, the focus is on *Mitleid* as compassion, as understood by Schopenhauer.

Envisaging compassion as a doubling of the ego, Nietzsche struggles to envisage a stable conception of self, or relation between self and other, that is not locked into either a rigid binary opposition between self and other – or into a monism where self is reduced to other or other is reduced to self. This position of Nietzsche in contrast with Schopenhauer will now be examined in spatial-relational terms as two contrasting projected structures of relation with regarding to understanding of *Mitleid*.

Compassion as concentric projected spatial structures of relation in contrast to egoism as diametric space – a spatial protolanguage of connection and the thick partition of separation

The problem of transcending egoism in *Mitleid* is one of finding a relation of assumed connection between self and other, which does not reduce one to the other; it is a challenge to traditional conceptions of an individual, self-contained self. Schopenhauer needs a raft to rescue a conception of self in compassion, which does not confuse self with other; concentric relational space of assumed connection moving from diametric oppositional space supplies this raft. Schopenhauer rejects the charge of Cassina that a person with compassion is 'deceived', stating that, 'it is precisely in his person, not in ours, that we feel the suffering, to our sorrow. We suffer *with* him and hence *in* him; we feel his pain as his, and do not imagine that it is ours' (OBM: 144/208f). Schopenhauer postulates a mode of being-*with* or being-*in*, which does not reduce self and other to a monistic relation, where one becomes the other.

This distinction between concentric spatialisation, as separation on the basis of assumed connection, and diametric opposition as assumed separation, can be directly uncovered from assumptions underlying a relational self, and relations between self and other, in Schopenhauer's *Mitleid*. The objections of Nietzsche et al. that Schopenhauer's description of compassion as, 'the immediate participation ... primarily in the suffering of another' (OBM: 144/208f) is mere egoism, are criticisms due to the projection of a diametric structure of relation onto Schopenhauer's way of thinking. It is the eschewal of monolithic projections of diametric spatial structures of opposition that is at issue.

Schopenhauer's following words on *Mitleid* can be reinterpreted in terms of offering an implicit model of concentric relation – of separation being on the basis of assumed connection between self and other – thereby leading to a path for rebuttal of the charge of egoism:

> As soon as this compassion is aroused, the weal and woe of another are nearest to my heart in exactly the same way, although not always in exactly the same degree, as otherwise only my own are. Hence the difference between him and me is now no longer absolute. (OBM: 144/208f)

As a common structural 'way' of assumed connection, the inner concentric circle is 'near' to the outer circle, while a degree of distance is maintained. Concentric spatialisation of relation resists collapse into a monistic fusion of identity, where the ego would assimilate the other's identity to its own. Furthermore, the dominion of this diametric structured mode of assumed separation, bringing an 'absolute' difference between self and other, is threatened by this mode of compassion, summoning a restructuring into concentric frames for experience. Concentric spatialisation expresses a conjoined relation between its mutually entwined poles to buttress the description of compassion of Schopenhauer as: 'We suffer *with* him and hence *in* him' (OBM: 147/211f). The concentric poles are 'in' one another and at a level of assumed connection 'with' the other. Compassion encounters the other in this structural sense as a relational state expressed through concentric space as assumed connection.

Compassion internalises the other as an extension of the self. This is a distinctive spatial-relational understanding of concentric assumed connection, where the inner circle of self extends to a second surrounding circle of the other. A different spatial structure of relation founds egoism, namely, a diametric oppositional spatial split between self and other, where the individual internalises the other with stark divisive boundaries of a diametric dualistic spatial relation.

Concentric spatial relation does not offer support for selflessness, for an obliteration of self that is also a target of Nietzsche's ire. Concentric space retains a sense of self through connection with each other. Thus, compassion is to be distinguished from selflessness, although sense of self here governing assumed connection between self and other is a preconscious state of assumed connection rather than a selfconscious state.[3]

Without having to accept crude labels of good and bad attributed in an essentialist manner to individuals, and recognising that Schopenhauer treats conceptions of good and bad as relative to the will,[4] Schopenhauer's wider point about different kinds of boundary between self and other offers a key insight:

> The bad man everywhere feels a thick partition between himself and everything outside him … The good character, on the other hand, lives in an external world that is homogenous with his own true being. The others are not non-I for him, but an 'I once more'. (OBM: 211)

This 'thick partition' of a diametric space of assumed separation contrasts with an assumed connection of common structure of relation to self and other in concentric relation; concentric relation treats the other as an extension of self rather that being a diametric split non-I from self. In a concentric relation of assumed connection, Schopenhauer's words are apposite: 'The suffering he sees in others affects him almost as much as his own … he *makes less of a distinction than is usually made between himself and others*' (WWRI: 399, italics in original).

This domain of relevance of modes of distinction for Schopenhauer, as differentiating membranes between self and other, can be directly expressed in spatial structural terms of concentric spatial relations to contrast with diametric spatial oppositions.

The rigid boundaries of division from other in egoism is again firmly expressed by Schopenhauer:

> However densely the mind of someone evil is enveloped in the *maya*, i.e., however firmly he is caught in the *principium individuationis*, seeing his own person as utterly distinct and separated from everyone else by a wide gulf (cognition that he firmly embraces, because it is the only viewpoint that will serve and support his egoism ...). (WWRI: 392)

Such a split assumed separation of diametric space framing the relation between self and other is reiterated by Schopenhauer, referring to 'the absolute barrier' (WWRI: 397) that is to 'present him as completely distinct from other individuals and divide him from these others and the countless miseries they suffer' (WWRI: 392). Such a diametric spatial veil is treated by Schopenhauer as being, in effect, a 'merely illusory nature of the *principium individuationis* and the distinction it posits between himself and others' (WWRI: 393). This egoistic mode is again treated as an illusory separation, 'the merely felt cognition of the illusoriness and the nothingness of the forms of representation that separate individuals' (WWRI: 393). Compassion overcomes this illusory diametric space between self and other to attune the person to a unitary will to life purportedly prior to space, time and causality. Compassion brings to an end, at least momentarily in the eternal present moment (as for Schopenhauer the past and future are illusory), the diametric spatial structures of egoism. The veil of space is this thick partition of diametric space.

It is to be emphasised that a concentric relation is not a monistic relation of identity so that the person would be the 'same' as the other; rather, as with the two poles of a concentric relation, allowance is made for a separation, although this separation is on the basis of an assumed connection. Focus on concentric spatio-relational aspects recognises an assumed connection that is not an excision of boundaries; rather it is a rendering of more fluid connective boundaries (than diametric structured opposition) that, nevertheless, retain distinction.

Janaway states that: 'Many will agree with Nietzsche that the doctrines about the One Will and the illusoriness of the individual are an excess and a mystical embarrassment' (2007: 63). This spatial framework challenges such a view, especially regarding the illusory dimension of the diametric spatial ego (although it does not go as far as maintaining the monistic position of Schopenhauer that 'the tormentor and tormented are one' (WWRI: 381)). Rather than being mere 'nonsense about compassion' as characterised by Nietzsche (GS: 153), Schopenhauer offers key distinctions about people's capacities to make distinctions between self and other; these can be concretised through specific spatial structures of relation, where diametric space is restructured and gives way to a prior relation of assumed connection in concentric spatial relation. The illusoriness of diametric spatial relations is not an excess; the thick walls of division underpinning diametric space can be opened and made transparent and permeable through concentric spatial connection.

Cajoling spatial assumptions out of the shadows of the tension between Schopenhauer's and Nietzsche's sharply opposing positions regarding compassion, the sense of mutuality is no vague intuition haunting relations between self and other. Rather it is a concrete relational space – of concentric space – mediating the internalisation of the other, the inclusion of the concrete other, as extension of the self. Mutuality in compassion brings an extension of boundaries from inner pole of self to outer pole surrounding the self, as extension of self to greet the other as an inside relation to self. This inside relation of assumed connection is not a reduction of self to other, or other to self.

It is notable that a major initiator of the debate on a protolanguage in European history, Étienne Bonnot, Abbé de Condillac (1715–1780), who published his 'Essay on the Origin of Human Knowledge' in 1746, focused on a dimension of experience that offers strong resonance with Schopenhauer's compassion:

> From this moment, he feels that he is eager to ease the other's pain, and he acts on this impression to the extent that it is within his ability. Thus by instinct alone these people asked for help and gave it. I say 'by instinct alone', for reflection could not as yet have any share in it. One of them did not say, 'I must bestir myself in that particular way to make the other understand what I need and to induce him to help me'; nor the other, 'I see by his motions that he wants to have something and I intend to give it to him'. But both acted as a result of the need that was most urgent for them. (Condillac 2001: 114–115)

However, this focus was not on a spatial protolanguage in relation to emotional–relational states such as compassion.[5] The interfused sense of concentric space needs to be brought to the fore.

Quintili interprets this account of Condillac as a pragmatic call to action as distinct from a phenomenological experience of assumed connection with the other:

> As in the case of Rousseau, who is often too sharply contrasted with Condillac, the Abbé recognizes the 'scream', that is the 'cry of the passions', which arises from the needs as the first source of speech production. The emphasis placed on 'pity', empathy, as we would say today, is very important to understand the pragmatic context in which we can place the theory of this 'language of action'. (2016: 39)

A spatial-phenomenology of experience must be distinguished from a pragmatic focus on action, while a spatial protolanguage offers resonance with a scrutiny of affective states, including in art, such as, for example, avant garde art.[6]

Nietzsche's alarming foreclosure of human possibility, of even a capacity for compassion, is shaped by his confinement within diametric spatial assumptions, of walls for experience that Schopenhauer would term a thick partition. Nietzsche's thick partition or 'hard skin' (GS: 103) only perceives the primordial rock, the primordial hardness to which he appeals; he only perceives the shell and not the yoke of the heart. Both Schopenhauer and Nietzsche reject the abstraction of Kant's categorical imperative as a fundamental injunction in moral terms, while sharing Kant's treatment of space as being merely phenomenal. Both reject the categorical imperative through recourse to prior experiential terrains, yet these terrains are themselves diametrically opposing ones. Whereas later Nietzsche invokes a prior experiential terrain of cruelty, Schopenhauer seeks the experience of compassion. It is tempting to characterise Nietzsche's cruelty as a diametric mirror image inversion of compassion. Nietzsche learns, at least indirectly from Schopenhauer, that morality is a projection of experience. However, a further step is needed. Experiences are projections of spaces, of concrete spatial structures.

Nietzsche's assault is on connection in compassion, where connection is an alien state and as if kindness were a crime or worse, a sheer mantra of manipulation. Compassion is treated, in effect, by Nietzsche as a meagre space not simply to be devoured by diametric space but as itself stillborn, unable to gain breath as a lived reality in human experience. The preying of diametric space guillotines connection, chilling connection into mere rivalry.

It is evident that Schopenhauerian compassion provides a challenge to traditional Western A/non-A diametric oppositions founding binary logic and conceptions of relation between self and other in diametric, Janus-faced terms. Schopenhauer's interest in Eastern culture, and notably Buddhism, is well known. Nietzsche, the self-styled antimoralist, even antiChrist of EH, the expounder of the antinomy between the Apollonian and Dionysian from BT onwards, is the propounder of diametric space *in extremis*. Schopenhauer's relational conception of compassion challenges traditional diametric structured Western logic, the framework within which his critics are embedded. His thought transcends this diametric structural mode of assumed separation between self and other.

Diametric space as illusion and obstacle

Janaway states that 'Schopenhauer carries "unselfing" to an extreme metaphysical pitch, where the self becomes both an illusion and an obstacle to true value' (2007: 58). It is to be noted that the lesser distinction between self and others as envisaged by Schopenhauer implies a continuity of self rather than simply being, as yet, a total selflessness of renunciation; on this reading, movement from diametric to concentric space in compassion is an intermediate stage, a transitional mediating state, a step on the way towards total selflessness of becoming at one with the will in itself.[7] While diametric space is both an illusory dimension considered from the vantage point of a prior experiential truth in concentric spatial relations of assumed connection, it is also an obstacle as resistance to concentric space. It is important also to acknowledge that in concentric space the self is sustained within the unitary whole of its relation to the other; it is the inner concentric pole in assumed connection with the other pole of the other as a concentric involved relation.

Concentric spatial relation is not an obliteration of self but a moistening of boundaries between self and other as a governing precondition for compassion. It is a restructuring of the diametric space constituting ego relations in the direction of concentric space. This restructuring is not so much an annihilation of egoistic experience but can be interpreted as a dissolution of the egoistic diametric space into the concentric realm. It is notable that Lévi-Strauss describes a difference between *destruction* and *dissolving* generally, which expresses a notion of inclusion in dissolving that is absent from sheer annihilation:

> [...] I believe the ultimate goal of the human sciences to be not to constitute, but to dissolve man ... I am not blind to the fact that the verb 'dissolve' does not in any way imply (but even excludes) the destruction of the constituents of the body subjected to the action of another body. The solution of a solid into a liquid alters the disposition of its molecules. It also often provides an efficacious method of putting them by so that they can be recovered in case of need and their properties be better studied. (1962: 247)

Shift from diametric structured oppositional space to concentric structured relational space of assumed connection involves a structural modification of the former but not its annihilation. It is to be recognised that at times Schopenhauer goes further than this 'less of a distinction', referring to abolition, 'the barrier between the I and the non-I is for the moment abolished' (OBM: 166), rather than the lessening of distinction through the assumed connection of concentric spatial relations, where the inner circle of self embraces the outer circle of other in a restructuring from a diametric oppositional split between self and other. The thick partition of the ice of diametric space gives way to the water of concentric space; these transitory boundaries are not sheer illusion as a nothingness but rather a limited vantage point of boundaries ripe for dissolution into a more expansive state of relations.

Compassion as renunciation or at least structural modification of ego is envisaged by Schopenhauer as part of a process of 'turning away', with a range of intermediate phrases such as 'voluntary renunciation, resignation, true composure and complete will-lessness' (WWRI: 406).[8] This passage offers implicit support for concentric spatial relations of assumed connection between self and other as a transitional space from egoism that compassion provides. Such concentric spatial relation does not offer succour for Schopenhauer's further position of complete will-lessness in renunciation. However, it does support Schopenhauer's shift away from abstract cognition (WWRI: 395–397) through compassion, where 'the cognition that gives rise to the negation of the will is intuitive and not abstract' (WWRI: 410).

The proposed spatial-relational shift for Schopenhauer's compassion in a process of movement from the obstacle of diametric space (as splits of assumed separation) to concentric spatial relations of assumed connection requires some modification of Schopenhauer's position. As a concentric *spatial* mode entering the movement from the realm of space, time and causality of empirical appearances, it is violating the excision of space from the realm of will as the Kantian *Ding-an-Sich* relied on for Schopenhauer's framework of metaphysics. Contrariwise, treated as a psychological rather than a metaphysical state, as a kind of intersubjective mode of relation, it moves compassion away from being exclusively in the realm of the unitary world of the will to life as a thing in itself. This latter movement is but a small step for Schopenhauer as he does at least in places imply recognition of compassion as existing in the phenomenal realm of appearances and cognition: '[C]ompassion is apparent in our heartfelt participation in the friend's well-being and woe' (WWRI: 403), 'cognition of other people's suffering, which is immediately intelligible from one's own suffering and the two are considered the same' (WWRI: 402).

Schopenhauer is seeking a basic orientation of openness to contrast with egoism, where a person 'takes as much interest in the sufferings of other individuals as he does in his own' and yet this goes further to include a capacity for a basic openness to suffering in life, to 'take upon himself the pain of the whole world' (WWRI: 405). Concentric openness of assumed connection as a precondition for compassion is not only an interpersonal state of relation, it is a capacity for experience of an existential pain.

For Schopenhauer, will is the essence of the world and 'the ultimate substrate of every appearance' (WN: 47/34). In Hübscher's words, Schopenhauer envisions the world as a will, which is unified, eternal and undivided, independent of space and time ('*einheitlich, ewig und ungeteilt, außerhalb von Raum und Zeit*') (1938: 15). In Schopenhauer's *Metaphysik der Natur*, a number of kinds of affect as dimensions of will are adumbrated (*Schreck, Freude, Schaam, Zorn, Furcht*) – and *Mitleid* is a notable omission. *Mitleid* differs from 'convulsions of the will' ("*Konvulsionen des Willens*") (MN: 75), and operates on a different level from the panoply of other affective states. Schopenhauer's conception of metaphysics is imbued with experience of suffering [*Leiden*] as key to discovering the world as 'will'. Richmond observes the connotation of suffering within the German term, *Mitleid*, literally suffering-with, in contrast to *Mitfreude*, literally, rejoicing-with (2004: 262).

Richmond highlights that a dedicated term for empathy in English was a translation from the German *Einfühlung*, which itself is quite a recent socio-historical construct, coined only in the early twentieth century. Thus, the term 'empathy' was unavailable to Schopenhauer and Nietzsche for their discussions of *Mitleid* (compassion). Empathy requires an object, whereas compassion is a wider background concept as a relational state; this echoes the distinction between fear and anxiety, where the former requires an object and the latter is a broader state of being for Heidegger (1927), building on Kierkegaard. Concentric relational space, as a precondition for compassion, opens a sense of some medium or membrane interfused, dwelling between self and other.

Compassion within the determinism of the empirical world: background conditions of space

Schopenhauer's reliance on Kant's Third Antinomy between freedom and causality, which places the phenomenal world under a mode of determinism with regard to the freedom of the noumenal will of Schopenhauer's will to life, invites the related question as to how compassion can exist in a determined causal dimension to move from the diametric space of egoism. In *On the Fourfold Root of the Principle of Sufficient Reason*, Schopenhauer criticises Kant's views on causality regarding inferences about succession with regard to empirical senses and judgment (FRP: 86) and on perception with regard to causality (FRP: 79). Nevertheless, across his work, Schopenhauer's understanding of freedom and causality holds firmly within the edifice of Kant's Third Antinomy with a transcendental realm of freedom at the level of the in itself and causal determinism in the realm of appearances. As Schopenhauer operates within a strict Kantian framework of transcendental freedom for the will to life as the thing in itself and determinism for the empirical world of appearances, he is committed to a view that: 'The person is never free, even though it is an appearance of a free will, because it is the already determined appearance of the free willing of that will' (WWRI: 315). This raises the question of compassion with respect to freedom and causality.

Compassion as a shift from diametric to concentric relational spaces must operate for Schopenhauer as a freedom through the will of the thing in itself, not through the diametric egoism of the phenomenal world as a cognitive choice as such. Although engaged cognitively with the suffering of the other person (WWRI: 402), compassion is precognitive and prerepresentational. Schopenhauer eschews mere intentionality for compassion: 'The old doctrine is that he *wills* what he cognizes; I say he *cognizes* what he wills' (WWRI: 319); 'entrance into freedom cannot be forced by any intention or resolution, but rather emerges from the innermost relation of cognition to willing in human beings' (WWRI: 432). Compassion is a metaphysical dimension, according to Schopenhauer. The question therefore arises as to how this spatial movement – from diametric spatial experience of egoism to concentric relational space of compassion that dissolves the rigid boundaries between self and other – pertains to the world of determinism in appearances.

A key starting point here is to recall Schopenhauer's emphasis on the negative, whether for happiness, satisfaction and its relation to pain; the pain or lack is primary and satisfaction is the overcoming of the lack (WWRI: 345–346). This focus on change as a negation process can also be applied to causality, as a focus on negating or at least changing supporting background conditions to change causal processes. An important passage in *The World as Will and Representation* develops this point:

> The only time this freedom can manifest itself directly in appearance … is when it brings to an end the thing that appears; and because the mere appearance … being a rung in the chain of causes, still continues to exist in time (which contains only appearances), it stands in contradiction to the will that manifests itself through this appearance, since the will negates what the appearance expresses. (WWRI: 430)

Mill's challenge to a clear-cut distinction between causal and non-causal states can shed light on the above point of Schopenhauer. Mill states:

> It is seldom if ever between a consequent and a single antecedent that this invariable sequence subsists. It is usually between a consequent and the sum of several antecedents the concurrence of all of them being requisite to produce, that is, to be certain of being followed by the consequent. (1872: 327)

Mill noted that one antecedent is very often termed the cause, the other antecedents being conditions. Actions that impact causally have hidden supporting conditions, without which the more obvious causal elements could not have occurred, just as striking a billiard ball to hit another presupposes the condition of gravitation. Causes necessarily operate within a background of supporting conditions that are structured sources of the cause's efficacy.

With regard to a movement within causal determinism, an implication of this insight is that change to background supporting conditions may shift the whole causal trajectory of a system. This need not be a destructive phenomenon; it may potentially be a constructive phenomenon, if the causal trajectories from the environment and egoism of the individual in space and time are destructive ones. In other words, a focus on changes to contingent or supporting background conditions may play a key role to undermine damaging causal trajectories of egoism.

If the background precondition for egoism of diametric structured oppositional space can be modified towards fostering other background supporting conditions of concentric space, this offers a key avenue for compassion within the deterministic empirical world of appearances. Diametric space can be brought to an end as a background condition for causal chains, to be replaced by a different background condition of concentric spatial relation. Schopenhauer's words are apt here: 'All that they can do is alter the direction of its striving, i.e., get the will to use a different path to search for the thing it invariably seeks' (WWRI: 321); concentric spatial relations is an altered direction of the striving of the diametric space of egoism, it is a structural modification of this diametric spatial movement of projection through the relative tension between contrasting modes of assumed connection and assumed separation. The 'rung in the chain of causes' recognised by Schopenhauer is somewhat malleable through their background spatial preconditions supporting causal impacts in the phenomenal world.

Concentric relational space of assumed connection framing experience of compassion is not itself a cognitive representation, at least not primarily. It is a precognitive, prerepresentational, taken-for-granted background mode of relation. This chapter has situated it as a mediating dimension between the empirical self of the *principium individuationis* and the will in itself in Schopenhaurian thought. Whether concentric space is part of the *Ding-an-Sich* of the will to life, as a microcosm of a wider systemic macrocosm of concentric structured relations, is beyond the scope of this argument. Nevertheless, suffice to observe that the specific Kantian framework of Schopenhauer would exclude any spatial notion from the realm of the *Ding-an-Sich*.

Compassion: a different kind of rationality

Janaway's introduction to the Cambridge edition of *The World as Will and Representation*, Volume I, characterises Schopenhauer's position as a shift away from the rational with regard to morality: 'The effective demotion of reason from any foundational role in characterizing human behaviour or explaining what has moral worth … [is one of the] notable distinguishing features of Schopenhauer's philosophy' (2010: xxiv). This arguably overstates Schopenhauer's position for compassion, if not renunciation; *Mitleid* is a shift from the rationalistic and abstraction that is not to be equated with the irrational. It is a different kind of reason that integrates with the emotional and relational.[9]

Schopenhauer's compassion is not mere irrationalism but a shift from decontextualised abstraction to relation as a basis for morality, through shifting of spatial-relational boundaries between self and other. With his pivotal conception of compassion, Schopenhauer is offering a different internalisation of the other from egoism. Compassion internalises the other as an extension of the self. This is a distinctive spatial-relational understanding of concentric assumed connection, where the inner circle of self extends to a second surrounding circle of the other. A different spatial structure of relation founds egoism, namely, a diametric oppositional spatial split between self and other, where the individual internalises the other with stark divisive boundaries of a diametric dualistic spatial relation. The lost scent of these spatial trajectories needs to be brought to the fore.

It is notable that concentric space extends the self (inner circle) into assumed connection with the other (outer circle), which allows for distinction of identity of self, while recognising fundamental connection to another and to the world (background space itself to the two concentric poles). Compassion is not egoism reformulated or doubled but a different kind of spatial-relation of the internalised other to self. Altering the direction of causal trajectories through change to malleable background spatial conditions as an interplay between diametric oppositional and concentric relational spaces, compassion can govern self–other relational frames, through modification of the diametric spatial precondition in the direction of concentric relational space for the internalisation of the other.

Taylor's words offer a limited vantage point on:

> [T]he domain of Schopenhauer, where our vital energy comes from a Will which is wild, unprincipled, amoral. This belief in our reliance on the forces of irrationality, darkness, aggression, sacrifice has become widespread in our culture; partly in the wake of Schopenhauer – say, with Nietzsche. (2007: 346)

This overlooks that Schopenhauer's compassion directly challenges a Nietzschean aggression and seeks a contextual mode of morality. The will to life for Schopenhauer is a blind force of striving and is in this sense premoral, a different level of description from anthropocentric concerns with morality.

This argument has not sought to enter the terrain of justifying why compassion is preferable to egoism, but rather to offer a pathway towards understanding how compassion can exist without being reducible to egoism, through a spatial framework for internalisation of the other in relation. The longstanding criticisms of Schopenhauer's conception of compassion (*Mitleid*) by critics that include Nietzsche, regarding compassion as basically egoism, need to be understood as an example of a diametric structured spatial projection of understanding and relation to other. This diametric space of assumed separation between self and other is not the only possible projected spatial structure, beyond a reductive monism that does not distinguish at all between self and other. Schopenhauer's account of compassion, across ample passages of text, highlights a preoccupation with a shift in relational boundaries between self and other, to overcome egoism through compassion. This shift can be understood as giving expression to a concentric spatial projection of understanding and relation, that lies in tension with a traditional Western A/non-A diametric structured logic of exclusion.

Schopenhauer's position on compassion is not only a highly tenable one against the backdrop of concentric relational space, it illustrates the distinctiveness of Schopenhauer's thought in challenging traditional Western taken for granted assumptions regarding relations between self and Other – and in replacing abstract cognition of morality with a fundamental relational mode of compassion.

Foreground–background interaction

Schopenhauer is seeking a basic orientation of openness to contrast with egoism, where a person 'takes as much interest in the sufferings of other individuals as he does in his own' and yet this goes further to include a capacity for a basic openness to suffering in life, 'take upon himself the pain of the whole world' (WWRI: 405). Concentric openness of assumed connection as a precondition for compassion is not only an interpersonal state of relation, it is a capacity for experience of an existential pain. A feature of concentric space observed by Lévi-Strauss is its interaction with background environment in a relation of relative openness in contrast to the relatively more closed structure of diametric space that does not interact with its background space. The point Schopenhauer makes here of the continuity in mode of relation between the assumed connection between self and other, and between self and pain of the world gains direct structural expression through concentric space as a duality of assumed connection between self and other. This concentric structure maintains its assumed connection also with the wider external background of the world, to take on the pain of assumed connection with the weight of the world.

Interestingly, without drawing on Schopenhauer here, Parkes (1994) observes a similar continuity in Nietzsche's Dionysian drive, where a common mode occurs between self and other, and self and world. However, as argued in Chapters 6 and 7, it is less a concentric space of assumed connection for Nietzsche, a concentric space that retains distinction through connection and rather a continuity as a more monistic fusion as unity. Parkes expands on different aspects of this as a monistic fusion, both interpersonally and with the natural world: 'The Dionysian drive dissolves the boundaries of the individual self in two ways: it breaks down the barriers separating it from other human selves, leading to a feeling of oneness with the social group or – by extension – with the human race; and it dissolves the boundaries between the individual human and the world of nature, conducing to a sense of unity with the cosmos' (1994: 67). This blissful annihilation is to be distinguished from ascetic negation of the will.

For Schopenhauer: 'The bad man everywhere feels a thick partition between himself and everything outside him ... The good character, on the other hand, lives in an external world that is homogenous with his own true being. The others are not non-I for him, but an "I once more"' (OBM: 211). This 'thick partition' of a diametric space of assumed separation contrasts with an assumed connection of common structure of relation to self and other in concentric relation; concentric relation treats the other as an extension of self rather that being a diametric split non-I from self. It is to be emphasised that Schopenhauer's point here is not only concerning a thick partition from self and other but also from 'everything outside him'; again he is pointing to the background space outside concentric dualism, the background of assumed connection with the external world in concentric space, as observed by Lévi-Strauss, a connection to the external background that is lost to the 'thick partition' of assumed separation between the diametric poles and their external background space. Schopenhauer's thick partition in the mode of orientation of the self to Other and world is a fundamental spatial recognition of the closure of diametric space in egoism.

Conceptions of foreground–background interaction are central to a well-known passage of Schopenhauer, cited also by Nietzsche in section 1 of *The Birth of Tragedy*:

> [T]rapped as he is in the *principium individuationis*, deceived by the veil of *maya*. – Just as a captain sits in a boat, trusting the weak little vessel as the raging, boundless sea raises up and casts down howling cliffs of waves; so the human individual sits calmly in a world full of sorrow, supported by and trusting in the *principium individuationis*, which is how the individual cognizes things as appearance. The boundless world, everywhere full of suffering, with its infinite past and infinite future, is alien to him – in fact it is a fairy tale: his vanishing little person, his unextended present, his momentary comfort, these alone have reality for him. (WWRI: 379)

Here, Schopenhauer's account of the closed structure of the boat is a metaphor for egoism as diametric spatial structures bringing noninteraction with the background space; this sealed mode of experience splits from awareness of the wider concentric expanding space. This invites further consideration of concentric space in relation to the world in itself, as a mediating or transitional space between the boat and sea, as well as giving expression to the boundlessness of the sea as the Schopenhauerian will in itself. It is notable from Schopenhauer's account that the background space within which the boat and also sea operate is excised from view and relevance; it is this background space mediating the relation between boat and sea that pertains to a domain of relevance for concentric space as a mediating space, a transitional dimension, between the will in itself and the *principium individuationis* of appearances.

Concentric space offers more permeable, transparent boundaries with the world, in contrast to the thick walled, opacity of diametric spatial structures. Schopenhauer gives expression to this contrast, stating that: 'The veil of *maya* has become transparent for this person, who is practised in works of love, and the delusion of the *principium individuationis* has deserted him' (WWRI: 400). Transparency and a movement of the veil of the thick walls of diametric space turns relations towards the increased permeability of concentric space; this concentric spatial relation underpinning compassion is intertwined with that of love. In the words of Schopenhauer, all love is compassion (WWRI: 401); both are held in the womb of concentric space.

This spatial-phenomenological approach can support Nietzsche's critique of selflessness, while firmly rejecting his critique of Schopenhauer's compassion (*Mitleid*). Concentric space as assumed connection between self and other, as internalisation of the other in the self as the expanded concentric pole of other in the self supports a capacity for compassion but this is one that does not vaporise the self, it does not eliminate the self as would the conception of selflessness. Nietzsche is on firmer ground if it is not compassion *per se* that is his main target but selflessness, loss of self, where self reduces to other in a monism that Nietzsche does not believe is possible. Nietzsche's more important assault is on a mode of selflessness. Concentric spatial relation between self and other retains and sustains the self in compassion. Space lurks and writhes within the assumption structure of the very terms of the disagreement between Schopenhauer and Nietzsche with regard to compassion.

Notes

1 Kant's categorical imperative is a mode of categorising. It is a category mode that breeds its claim for universality. Yet such a categorising mode is far from being primordial but derives from prior spatial-experiential modes of relation, diametric and concentric space. As projections of experience into thought and morality, these spaces offer malleable yet durable preconditions for assumptions that give 'grounds' to truth claims resting on categories. The mode of abstracting in categorisation, rests on spatial experiential projections that presuppose notions such as containment, inclusion and exclusion (see also Lakoff and Johnson 1980).

2 See Janaway (2007) for an account of these objections of Nietzsche, including a view in Nietzsche's BGE that by placing compassion for suffering as key to morality, Schopenhauer gives preference to what is passive and vulnerable in people, rather than human's strength and creativity. For an account of advantages of compassion, see Wolf (2015).

3 See the argument in Chapter 4 that concentric space is prior to subject–object distanciation founding selfconsciousness, and is a prerepresentational state of relation.

4 'This concept [of good] is essentially relative, and designates the suitability of an object to any particular effort of the will. So anything that is agreeable to the will in any one of its expressions, that is conducive to its purpose, is intended in the concept of good' (WWRI: 387).

5 For Quintili: 'The conclusion of Condillac's Essay is not far from the philosophical statement that will later be the main thesis of Rousseau: passions (fear, joy, sexual desire, hatred etc.) drive the process of development of the signs system of a primitive language towards ever greater precision.' Later, Condillac changes his ideas about this topic, with his *Grammaire* (1775), in accordance with the thesis about the analogy to and the imitation tools of natural language. Nevertheless, the main difference between Rousseau and Condillac is that, according to the latter, such a language consists, primarily (but not exclusively), of bodily actions and not of articulated sounds' (2016: 39).

6 See, for example, Boguska-Kawałek (2014) on protolanguage developed as a reaction of individuals to the stimuli of the environment, and, along with all sorts of non-verbal means, facilitated them the expression of affective states of their mind. She

argues that certain parallels can be noticed between the beliefs concerning human protolanguage and the demands on the means of expression in art, its mission, and goals formulated by members and theorists of the avant garde movement. However, a spatial protolanguage is not necessarily as a reaction to environment.

7 See also Janaway (2007) on compassion as a step on the way to renunciation.

8 As Shapsay and Ferrell observe: 'Schopenhauer's system is in general characterized by degrees (e.g., he talks of grades of the manifestation of the metaphysical will captured by the doctrine of the Ideas; grades of insight into the metaphysical reality – in aesthetic experience, compassion and resignation – and these correspond to degrees of will-lessness' (2015: 65).

9 See also Downes' (2012, 2015) reinterpretation of Gilligan's (1982) frames for moral reasoning in spatial-relational terms that challenge a logic of abstraction through a focus on an ethic of care. Compassion can be envisaged as a key background state of relation, as a trajectory guiding moral choices, through framing moral problems in terms of connection between self and other, as through examples of care, offered by Gilligan (1982).

References

Bobko, A., *Schopenhauers Philosophie des Leidens*. Würzburg: Königshausen & Neumann, 2001.

Boguska-Kawałek, J., 'The Discourse of Avant-Garde Art as an Expression of Primordial Emotions of Man'. In P. P. Chruszczewsk, J. R. Rickford, K. Buczek, A. R. Knapik and J. Mianowski (eds.), *Ways to Protolanguage 3*. Wrocław: Wyższa Szkoła Filologiczna we Wrocławiu & Polska Akademia Nauk, 2014.

Cartwright, D. E., 'Compassion and Solidarity with Sufferers: The Metaphysics of Mitleid', *European Journal of Philosophy*, 2008, 16: 292–310.

Condillac, E.-B. de, *Essay on the Origin of Human Knowledge*, H. Aarsleff (ed.). Cambridge: Cambridge University Press, 2001.

D'Aquili, E., 'The Influence of Jung on the Work of Claude Lévi-Strauss', *Journal of the History of the Behavioral Sciences*, 1975,11): 41–48.

Downes, P., *The Primordial Dance: Diametric and Concentric Spaces in the Unconscious World*. Oxford/Bern: Peter Lang, 2012.

Downes, P., 'Developing Derrida's Psychoanalytic Graphology: Diametric and Concentric Spatial Movements' , *Derrida Today*, 2013,6(2): 197–221.

Downes, P., 'Diametric and Concentric Spatial Structures Framing Belief Systems', *Cybernetics and Systems*, 2015,46(6–7): 510–524.

Gilligan, C., *In a Different Voice*. Cambridge, MA: Harvard University Press, 1982.

Heidegger, M., *Being and Time*. Trans. J. MacQuarrie and E. Robinson. Oxford: Basil Blackwell, 1927/1962.

Hübscher, A., 'Arthur Schopenhauer: Leben und Lehre', in *Festschrift 1788–1938 zum 150. Geburtstage von Arthur Schopenhauer Gedentfeiern in seiner Geburtstadt Danzig vom 21–26 Februar 1938*. Danzig: Senat der Freien Stadt Danzig, 1938.

Janaway, C., *Beyond Selflessness: Reading Nietzsche's Genealogy*. Oxford: Oxford University Press, 2007.

Janaway, C., 'Introduction to Arthur Schopenhauer', in *The World as Will and Representation*, Volume 1 Trans. J. Norman, A. Welchman and C. Janaway. Cambridge: Cambridge University Press, 2010.

Lakoff, G. and Johnson, M., *Metaphors We Live By*. Chicago, IL: University of Chicago Press, 1980.
Lévi-Strauss, C., *The Savage Mind*. Trans. G. Weidenfeld. Nicolson Ltd. Chicago, IL: University of Chicago Press, 1962.
Mill, J. S., 'A System of Logic', in R. F. McRae (ed.). *Collected Works*, Vol. VII, Books I, II, III. Toronto: University of Toronto Press, 1872/1973.
Morioka, M., 'Commentary: Constructing Creative Appropriations', *Culture & Psychology*, 2007, 13: 189–196.
Parkes, G., *Composing the Soul: Reaches of Nietzsche's Psychology*. Chicago, IL: University of Chicago Press, 1994.
Quintili, P., 'ThePrehistory of Protolanguage's Notion. Condillac, Rousseau, De Brosses and the Origins of Language in the Eighteenth Century', in Theoria et Historia Scientaiarum, Vol. XIII. Toruń: Nicolaus Copernicus University, 2016.
Richmond, S., 'Being in Others: Empathy from a Psychoanalytical Perspective', *European Journal of Philosophy*, 2004,12: 244–264.
Shapshay, S. and Ferrell, T., 'Compassion or Renunciation? That Is the Question of Schopenhauer's Ethics', *Enrahonar*, 2015, 55: 51–69.
Taylor, C., *A Secular Age*. Boston, MA: Harvard University Press, 2007.
Wolf, U., 'How Schopenhauer's Ethics of Compassion can Contribute to Today's Ethical Debate', *Enrahonar*, 2015, 55: 41–49.
Young, J., *Schopenhauer*. London/New York: Routledge, 2005.

Chapter 4

Rapture and space

Rapture as an experiential expansion in Dionysian music: tentative Nietzschean steps towards concentric space as opened boundaries in his gloss on Schopenhauer's *principium individuationis*

Throughout the *Birth of Tragedy*, Nietzsche is engaged in a quest for a life force, as a life principle associated with the Dionysian, with 'the glowing life of Dionysian enthusiasts' (BT: 22). Engaging with 'the Dionysian life' (BT: 110) as 'pulsating life, pain and pleasure' (BT: 100), he associates life with movement, as 'urgency' 'continual movement' (BT: 49). As part of a life principle, a fundamental insight of Nietzsche's BT is the importance of an experiential movement of expansion from a more rigidly boundaried state, an opening that he perceives in Dionysian terms as immersion with a universal language of music prior to representation. The current spatial-phenomenological questioning of rapture is less concerned with its pertinence to aesthetic experience than with its fundamental importance as expression of a life dimension.

Music is for the Nietzsche of BT,[1] 'an unmediated copy of the will itself' (BT: 88), 'the unmediated language of will' (BT: 89), where he associates the will itself in Schopenhauerian terms as a will to life principle. This is not to state that Nietzsche attributes this to all kinds of music. He also refers to 'masked imitation music' (BT: 62), 'alienated' music (BT: 105), thus opening a horizon for life as alienation, as subject to an alienating process.

Elsewhere, Nietzsche reiterates the role music is purported to play in an experiential expansion in direct lived experience, 'the sovereignty of music, as Schopenhauer understood it ... the language of the will itself, speaking straight out of the abyss as its most personal, original, and direct manifestation' (GM: 72). On this account, a living melody of rapture sought by Nietzsche through music inspires a restructuring of experience towards an intimate engagement with a life dimension, through unmediated contact in the moment with the will itself.

Early Nietzsche seeks a universal language (of music) prior to language and sets out counterpoles (Dionysian and Apollonian) in terms of relative differences as part of a complementary interplay. The question arises as to whether this experiential shift as opening can be interpreted in terms of an interplay between diametric and concentric spaces, specifically regarding contrasts between the relative closure divorcing from interaction with background in diametric spatial systems compared with the relative openness assuming connection to background environment in concentric spatial systems, outlined in Chapter 2.

This core spatial structural movement between relative openness and closure arguably underpins a pivotal feature of Nietzsche's understanding of the Dionysian mode of experience, as a life principle, at least in aesthetic terms. This major feature of early Nietzsche's understanding of the Dionysian draws explicitly from Schopenhauer's account of the *principium individuationis* in his account of a will to life principle. Both Nietzsche's and Schopenhauer's positions here require further excavation in spatial terms.

A centrepiece of Nietzsche's argument to bridge the Dionysian myth with that of Schopenhauer's will to life is his treating of the Apollonian as the *principium individuationis* giving boundaries and form to the Dionysian will to life. Schopenhauer's account of a man caught in the veil of *maya* is applied by Nietzsche to the Apollonian:

> As a sailor sits in a small boat in a boundless raging sea, surrounded on all sides by heaving mountainous waves, trusting to his frail vessel; so does the individual man sit calmly in the middle of a world of torment, trusting to the *principium individuationis*. (WWRI: 379)

The closed boundaried vessel of the ship seeks to shut out the vast infinity of expansion beyond itself, just as diametric spatial structures operate as a closure sealed off from the wider background beyond. As Lévi-Strauss observes, the relatively closed structure of diametric relations contrasts with the relative openness and expansion for interaction with background of concentric structured relations. The illusion of totality of Schopenhauer's ship, of Nietzsche's Apollonian mode, through remaining fixed within the tight boundaries of diametric space, all gives way to a more fundamental reality of the more expansive background, the wider raging sea of stimuli and what Nietzsche characterises as the Dionysian force for experience entwined with a life principle.

Schopenhauer's *principium individuationis* sets the scene for an understanding in terms of an interplay between concentric and diametric spaces. The sailor in the boat does not engage with the storms of the ocean beyond, which engulf the whole background to the boat; he or she operates in a defensive diametric spatial systemic mode of interaction with the background environment – as a 'closed system' (Lévi-Strauss 1963: 152) of assumed separation from background, as a splitting from engagement with the storms of stimuli. Schopenhauer apprehends this mode of closure, as a foreclosure of a different possibility, namely, of a relative opening to the more fundamental reality of the stormy seas. The narrow firmness of the boat's solidity is but a frail buttress against the vast expanse of fluidity of storms and ocean. The diametric spatial mode of closure, of resting within this frail vessel of diametric boundaried space, obscures the experiential truth of the wider reality. Schopenhauer and subsequently Nietzsche challenge the sealed diametric mode of existence, this illusion of closure in the veil of *maya*.

The importance of Schopenhauer's *principium individuationis* in Nietzsche's thought has frequently been neglected by commentators seeking to examine the influence of Schopenhauer on Nietzsche. For example, this aspect of Schopenhauer's thought is completely overlooked in Copleston's (1942/1975) account of their interrelation. Moreover, the closest Kaufmann comes to scrutiny of the relation between Schopenhauer's *principium individuationis* and Nietzsche is in Kaufmann's interrogation of Nietzsche in relation to romanticism which identifies 'the basic distinction … between two states of being: the "overfulness of life" and the "impoverishment of life", power and impotence' (1975: 375). This analysis does not develop Schopenhauer's insight in fundamentally spatial terms. However, overfulness of life implicitly rests on spatially imbued assumptions, as the monistic fusion with the swirling background storms and sea; impoverishment of life is the retreat into the diametric spatial closure for experience, through a mode of confinement of horizons to the boundaries of the frail vessel of Schopenhauer's boat. Kaufmann, in effect, constructs these two states of being, monistic fusion and diametric closure, as being themselves in a diametric mirror image inverted relation of power versus impotence.

Nietzsche borrows this pivotal insight of Schopenhauer regarding a fundamental experiential interplay between closure and openness to powerful dynamic background stimuli, elevating it into a key hallmark of the Dionysian, as an additional mediating limb of a will to life principle.[2] Schopenhauer's insight is not merely metaphorical but resides within prior primordial spatial structures of relation. Nietzsche's reworking of Schopenhauer's account in Dionysian terms is an attempt to render concrete a mode of rapture or ecstasy, a primordial *ekstasis* in an experiential dynamic life opening beyond rigid boundaries of experience. Schopenhauer's metaphorical account gives expression to the archetypal spatial contrast and movement between the relative closure of diametric space and the relative openness with background of concentric space.

It is significant that Nietzsche's recourse to a Dionysian dimension to dismantle the Apollonion *principium individuationis* strays far from historical accuracy here regarding the Dionysian. Whereas Kerenyi highlights some disparities between a Nietzschean account of Dionysus and the historical evolution of the Dionysian myth in antiquity, it is for this passage of Nietzsche, reliant on Schopenhauer, that Kerenyi reserves most of his disdain. This kernel of Nietzsche's Dionysian experience, 'Dionysian enchantment', is trenchantly criticised in Kerenyi's authoritative historical account of the Dionysian in ancient Greece, as where Nietzsche's 'account becomes a fairy tale':

> Now, with the gospel of universal harmony, each one feels himself not only united, reconciled, and fused with his neighbour, but as one with him, as if the veil of *maya* had been torn aside and were now merely fluttering in tatters before the mysterious primordial unity. (1976: 135)

Kerenyi's more strictly historical account of the Dionysian myth in ancient Greece supports many of the core theses of Nietzsche regarding the Dionysian in BT. Kerenyi affirms the Dionysian sacrificial rite as one of the basic facts of Greek religious history, with the 'differentiated' (1976: 52) Dionysian myth still retaining a common core including a definite well-ordered feature of association with wine and a dual aspect of life and death. He questions Nietzsche's wish to claim all intoxication for Dionysus (1976: 136), although he accepts that the historical relation of Dionysus to wine was 'definite and well ordered' (1976: 76). A key dimension of this is intoxication as a shift out of self-consciousness to a more immediate level of relation to the experiential moment, as a lubrication out of boundaried perception, including shifts from habits of self-perception.

The closest Kerenyi comes to supporting Nietzsche's view of music as a suspension of Apollonian boundaries, through a movement from the closure of the *principium individuationis*, is in his portrayal of spirit: '"spirit" is openness and expansion of vision, a primordial experience of man. Openness and expansion arise naturally from a gift peculiar to man' (1976: 7). Kerenyi's description is tantamount to a succinct account of relative openness of concentric spatial systems compared to diametric spatial systems' closed boundaries; this is an extending and not shattering of boundaries of awareness, 'this Dionysian area of suspended boundaries, where the world was not the limited world of men but a *world of life shot through with spirit*' (Kerenyi 1976: 341) (italics in original).[3]

While one key question is with regard to what is filtered out from Nietzsche's account of the Dionysian myth, the opposite question will be considered here for current purposes – how Nietzsche has embellished the Dionysian myth beyond the historical facts, so that the revealing projection from Nietzsche of emotional excess on the Dionysian itself can itself offer some phenomenological insights for structural features of lived experience. Nietzsche later concedes in *Ecce Homo* that the Apollo and Dionysus of BT is about his own personal experiences (EH: 65). Cognisant of Nietzsche's recognition that 'every great philosophy' is an 'unconscious auto-biography' (BGE: 4), space is being viewed as a surreptitious projection of Nietzsche's experience, an unconscious autobiography of the contours of his experiential capacities and scope.

Kerenyi's characterisation of Nietzsche's Dionysian enchantment as mere fairy tale requires further exploration. Developing his explication of enchantment, Kerenyi quotes Pausanias 'the Thyiades swarm in a trance for Dionysus and Apollo' (1976: 224). Thus, even Apollo is associated with trances. Again Kerenyi refers to 'her trance ... which endured by daylight under the sign of Apollo ... she trembled in her cold ecstasy ... after becoming one with her god Apollo' (1976: 229). This offers at least a *prima facie* challenge to a view of the Apollonian as the *principium individuationis* to be dismantled by Dionysian rapture (although later Nietzsche recognises Apollonian trances). It is not a denial of Dionysian trancelike ecstasy for which Kerenyi provides supportive evidence; neither is it a denial of associations of Apollo with order and harmony. However, association of trancelike states with the Apollonian requires that the early Nietzschean version of the Apollonian be cut from a cloth that is not only selective, at best; it denies common overlapping features between the Dionysian and Apollonian regarding purportedly key distinguishing dimensions of each pole, such as that of ecstatic enchantment as the sole preserve of the Dionysian.

Kerenyi views Nietzsche as having yoked together Schopenhauer's will to life and a Dionysian life principle into a somewhat uneasy synthesis, particularly in the account of music and the *principium individuationis*. Yet some key common features pervade both, for example, the experiential opening as a shift out of a selfconscious mode of experience of a strongly boundaried self into a state of enchantment, rapture or at least intoxication that also involves an unseating of selfconscious experience, as if into a prior more primary mode of experience.

Nietzsche's Dionysus life principle must be viewed as an excess on the historical. It is not only a typical Nietzschean excess but also one needing interpretation fundamentally in spatial terms, as projected structures of primordial experience. Nietzsche's gloss on the historical Dionysus myth does not arrive *ex nihilo*, but rather as a specific primordial experiential projection of spatially mediated experience.

Nietzsche's account of the expansion of awareness beyond the *principium individuationis* can be interpreted not simply as historical error but also as being most revealing of his own projected experience onto the Dionysian myth. Here boundaries are to be suspended and a primordial openness is to be extended not shattered. Is it in this very fluidating rapture and enchantment that Nietzsche attains a recognition of concentric spatial experience?

The diametric boundaries and walls of the individual as frail vessel in Nietzsche's interpretation of Schopenhauer's *principium individuationis* cannot house the expanding space of the Dionysian. Nietzsche seeks an alternative site for experience than the confines of the closure of the isolated individual, the illusion of the split self in the *maya* of the *principium individuationis*. Is this expanded space a quest for concentric flowing dimensions of experience?

The issue of crossing in experience from foreground to background space: a protolanguage of monism, concentric spatial relation and diametric spatial opposition

With his *principium individuationis*, Schopenhauer has arguably inaugurated a tradition, at least in Western thought,[4] of preoccupation with foreground–background interaction in terms of opening and closure.[5] This lineage can be traced through Nietzsche's quest for a musical opening from boundaried Apollonian experience to the abyss of the background storms in the Dionysian as part of 'the eternal wound of life' (BT: 96), to Freud's (1920) economic principle of tension reduction seeking to manage a level of acceptable stimuli for apprehension, to Munch's background swirling storms as a primal scream through the universe that cannot be escaped from, even on the foreground bridge, to Lévi-Strauss' recognition of diametric structured systems as a relative closure from background; it embraces Plath's *Bell Jar* and Fromm's fear of freedom, fear of an opening to a vast fluid storms of possibilities that engulf the individual and prompt a retreat into closure. Plath's journals of 1952 offered an experiential account of an opening from the closure of the bell jar in anticipation of her later work:

> It is like lifting a bell jar off a securely clockworklike functioning community, and seeing all the little busy people stop, gasp, blow up, and float in the inrush (or rather outrush) of the rarified scheduled atmosphere – poor little frightened people, flailing impotent arms in the aimless air. That's what it feels like: getting shed of a routine … one feels uncomfortable when jounced out of the repetitive rut. (Plath 1952, in Wagner 2000: 39)[6]

While all these concerns coalesce around a range of responses of opening and closure to a vast background, it is Lévi-Strauss and Munch who engage with this existential dilemma uniquely in spatial-structural terms, expanding on Schopenhauer's[7] and subsequently Plath's accounts in pictorial terms. It is also arguable that Munch, like Lévi-Strauss, uncovered this dilemma in explicit spatial-structural terms of concentric and diametric space (Downes 2012) in his iconic painting *The Scream*. Lévi-Strauss offered not only a concretisation of this dilemma in spatial-structural terms but also an expansion of the breadth of its relevance to cross-cultural contexts, building on the observations of other anthropologists, *although without an existential or phenomenological focus*.

Nietzsche's account is notable for two structural features – first, his account of *opening is a violent one, based on annihilation* of this relatively closed boundaried structure, which is to be torn open, broken, burst, 'tearing asunder of the *principium individuationis*' (BT: 25), 'annihilation of the veil of *maya*' (BT: 26), 'burst apart' (BT: 86). It is not an account of fluidly dissolving such boundaries, or melting them into a wider concentric kind of space. It is a matter of vaporising and annihilating this structure, not modifying it.

For Nietzsche, 'the eternal life of the will remains untouched by this annihilation' (BT: 90). It is not a transformative dissolving into the will. This experiential restructuring offers an 'annihilation of the usual limits and borders of existence' (BT: 46). Nietzsche clearly seeks an expansion beyond diametric space. What is not clear is the spatial structure underpinning that sought for expansion. It is a purported expansion as annihilation, as obliteration of boundaries, so that Nietzsche's quest is for no boundaries, no mediating space with the infinity of stimuli, with the vast ocean's storms.

Second, another notable structural feature is the counterpoint to this boundaried Apollonian *principium individuationis* as one of a *monistic fusion* with the will in itself, as the Dionysian counterpole. The Apollonian is 'the apotheosis of the *principium individuationis*' (BT: 31), as a 'drawing boundaries' against 'the sudden surge of the Dionysian tide' (BT: 58). The Dionysian is a hurling fast into an overwhelming force where the individual is dismantled; no semblance of individual identity is to be retained or expressed in this Dionysian fusion, 'the joy experienced in the annihilation of the individual … the Dionysian art which gives expression to the will in its omnipotence as it were behind the *principium individuationis*' (BT: 90).

Not only is the veil of *maya* to be obliterated, individual identity in experience is to be dismantled in 'orgiastic self-annihilation' (BT: 115). This is a *monistic* fusion that is significantly a challenge to selfconscious experience as primary and is further illustrated where Kerenyi quotes Muller, as: 'Nature overpowering the mind and hurrying it out of a clear selfconsciousness (whose most perfect symbol is wine) lies at the basis of all Dionysian creations' (1976: 27). Nietzsche's description is similarly of 'an overpowering feeling of unity which leads back to the heart of nature' (BT: 45), 'mystical self-abandonment and unity' (BT: 36). This again leaves no sense of retention of a restructured identity of the individual in connection as in concentric space and treats unity in monistic terms as fusion. Individual identity is annihilated, abandoned, overpowered through the fusion of this monism, a fusion with nature and potentially interpersonally with other people. Parkes observes the danger of fusion with a primal one, where a vaporising of all boundaries brings a collapse into all the figures in history (1994: 74–75), echoing Nietzsche's own personal collapse. This fusion reveals not only a dismantling of the hard borders of diametric spatial boundaries for experience but also a lack of the more porous, permeable concentric boundaries for a more fluid, dynamic engagement with the infinity of background stimuli.

Fusion into background may take place at an individual level of experience in relation to a drowning in the round ocean of external stimuli, bringing a loss of individual awareness. Another version, although it is far from being the sole or dominant version of this, is a subsuming of individual identity into the group in the collective Dionysian ritual. The Dionysian can be interpreted as both a collective ritual and a structure of individual experience. As a collective ritual, the fusion in the Dionysian is with the crowd, as a collective conformity that is to be distinguished from an individual experiential restructuring.

Some aspects of Nietzsche's account point tentatively towards an opening and loosening that is more resonant with concentric space as a structure of individual experience, where he invokes the *principium individuationis* explicitly, referring to 'loosening of the chains of the individual' (BT: 111) as a mode of experience that 'lies open' (BT: 86). A life principle as an experiential *dynamis*, as a foundational restructuring in experience to move towards a more intense apprehension of the present moment, offers a connective openness that faces (and dissolves) pain. It also offers affinity with Byron's celebration of a life intensity in *Childe Harold's Pilgrimage* 'from the high host/Of stars to the lulled lake and mountain-coast/All is concentred in a life intense'.

Early Nietzsche invokes a mode of original pain, 'the Dionysian musician is himself wholly and exclusively original pain and original echo of that pain' (BT: 35). This opening and loosening of boundaries offers here some concentric imagery, the concentric echo. This recognition of an original primordial pain, also described by Nietzsche as 'the eternal wound of life' (BT: 96), invites comparison with Schopenhauer's understanding of a basic openness to other in compassion as resting on an experiential capacity for being open to the pain of the world. The concentric spatial relation of self with other is, implicitly for Schopenhauer, contingent on a prior background concentric mode of opened connection to background. Nevertheless, despite these concentric spatial hints and fragrances, this central concept for Nietzsche with regard to an experiential openness is one of monistic fusion as sheer obliteration of boundaries. In other words, there is no substantial scope for an embedded connection of intensity in the Dionysian as the will to life; there is no capacity or vision of a concentric spatial relation of openness as assumed connection with background. Not only is space rendered redundant and ephemeral, following both a Kantian and Schopenhauerian orthodoxy regarding the in-itself that is to be non-spatial, the individual is to be transposed into a will to life domain that requires complete surrender of his or her identity. With regard to the axis of opening versus closure, Nietzsche's opening as fusion with a totality does not encompass a concentric spatial opening, although he recognises the need to open beyond diametric space.

This monistic quest for no spatial relation beyond total fusion must be clearly distinguished as a mode of experience, as a structure of experiential space, from a concentric spatial relation of assumed connection with the vast background stimuli, a connection and interaction that is not annihilation or obliteration of identity. This intoxication as obliteration of self, as annihilation of boundaries, whether wine fuelled or through other intoxicatory substances such as hallucinatory drugs, is to be distinguished from the rapturous opening of concentric spatial structured experience.

The prerepresentative mode of music as a concentric spatial dimension restructuring experience

Nietzsche sought to go beyond subject–object based experience in Dionysian music, stating that the subject–object distinction is 'completely irrelevant to aesthetics' (BT: 38). Challenge to the observer-observed imports a level of experience prior to the image, where in the 'imageless' Dionysian art of music (BT: 19), there is 'no need for the image and the concept' (BT: 41); it is prior to language (BT: 42) and enters a level of experience of 'original suffering ... devoid of image and concept' (BT: 35). Going to a level prior to signification, Nietzsche is also seeking a mode of experience prior to image based division into subject–object dualisms.[8] To see an image, a perceiving subject and object or image is required to sustain a space of assumed separation, what Ricoeur (HHS) terms a *distanciation* between subject and object. *This distanciation is an assumed separation of diametric space.* Thus, Nietzsche is seeking a space *prior to* such diametric spatial divisions into subject and object, perceiver and image. Again early Nietzsche's search is for an embedded beyond, beyond diametric space – both beyond closure and beyond the assumed separation as a relational precondition for the subject–object distinction.

Interpreting, with Davey (1991), BT as a response to a predicament of existential meaningless,[9] Nietzsche's construction of the Dionysian is for a distinct existential purpose that treats the historical as a means to a wider narrative and end.[10] In contrast, Kerenyi seeks to construe the Dionysian historically on its own terms. Accepting Davey's recognition that Nietzsche's task was not sheer historical reconstruction, as applied to the Dionysian myth, the points of divergence from history become not weaknesses but of renewed existential-phenomenological interest for interpreting Nietzsche's argument. It is notable that Nietzsche links Zarathustra explicitly to Dionysus: '*But that is the concept of Dionysian himself*' (E: 73). In his later thought, Zarathustra is a repository for the features Nietzsche projects onto the Dionysian myth without having to have much recourse to historical accuracy. Although also rooted loosely in the history of Zardusht or Zarathustra, known to the ancient Greeks as Zoroaster, the Persian prophet, who lived around 1000BC, if not before (Frankopan 2015), he steps with Zarathustra beyond even the poetic licence of interpretation of Dionysus where he added his own projections such as the annihilation of the *principium individuationis*.

Zarathustra offers echoes of the pre-perceptual emphasised in the Dionysian of BT. In Parkes' words: 'Zarathustra claims that any knowledge gained through pure perceiving – obsessed with eliminating all traces of will and desire in order chastely to receive and, coolly moonlike, to reflect reality – will be sterile and barren' (1994: 236), Zarathustra 'accuses the pure perceivers of wanting to touch the beauty of the earth only with their eyes' (1994: 237).

Whereas some commentators emphasise Nietzsche's concern with mystical states of rapture (e.g., Bataille 1945;[11]Stambaugh 1994), current concerns are not to examine any such spatial-structural rapture as concentric spatial experience in relation to beauty as such in art. This spatial interrogation of rapture is as a potentiality for life experience. This potentiality for an intensification of joy in existence may be as an *ongoing* experiential mode of relation or as a momentary state, as Bataille (1945) claims is typically the sole experiential possibility for rapture.

Stambaugh suggests on the basis of passages from Zarathustra that a key dimension of *das Fremde* (the foreign, the Other) may have been mystical experience (1994: 9). The current argument places this mystical experiential concern earlier in Nietzsche's thought regarding experiential apprehension of music as rapture or bliss. For Stambaugh's 'the other Nietzsche', 'the German word for "strange" here, *fremd*, indicates that Zarathustra has been in a state completely foreign and other to his normal way of experiencing' (1994: 24). A shift occurs in the experiential centre of gravity, from the distanciation of assumed separation constructing the subject–object boundaries to an assumed connection prior to these experiential boundaries.

Concentric spatial connection between its poles is prior to the distanciation of the assumed separation built into the subject–object dualism and hence is prior to experience as intentionality that requires an object of experience. It is prior to selfconsciousness as it does not include a distance where the self would be an object for the self to perceive. It is a pre-perceptual, pre-subject/object mode of experience offering an immediacy to awareness that Nietzsche may have been seeking to express through his notion of music as the unmediated will to life. This cessation of cognition invokes a prior mode of bliss, a rush of rapture in the heightened assumed connection of concentric space.

Taking seriously Nietzsche's concerns with imageless and preconceptual experience, illustrated through a purportedly universal language of music, concentric space can be interpreted as a movement from diametric spatial preconditions for Apollonian image-based boundaried experience. In other words, concentric space serves as at least a potential direction towards which Nietzsche seeks to leap, to challenge and restructure the everyday visual diametric boundaried experience of the Apollonian into an accelerated concentric spatial movement prior to selfconsciousness. Selfconsciousness is supported by the precondition of assumed separation given by diametric space.

A central tenet of romanticism for Berlin is 'to raise everybody to some passionate level of self-expressive experience, of such a kind as perhaps only divinities, in older works of literature, were supposed to manifest' (2000: 146).[12] This is pivotal to the ecstatic opened boundaries of concentric space in the overcoming of diametric spatial boundaries of the *principium individuationis*. In this dimension, it could be said that Nietzsche offers a romantic vision of music as an opening of pre-image-based experience.[13] Again there are echoes of Byronic themes, in *Childe Harold's Pilgrimage*: 'Then stirs the feeling infinite, so felt/In solitude, where we are least alone/A truth which through our being there doth melt/And purifies from self; it is a tone/The soul and source of music.' It is an amplification of awareness that for many of the romantics is available for everyone, at least potentially, although Nietzsche retreats into a more elitist view of this experiential domain.

It is not a matter of leaving diametric space to long decay as a colossal wreck but rather of its restructuring, its structural modification into concentric space. The expansion of experience through rapture offers an antidote to drowning in the *taedium vitae* of a fraught selfconsciousness. It offers a spontaneity that embraces the moment and undoes a displacement from the moment in the dividing walls of diametric space, a dividing membrane not only of self from Other, of self from environment but also undoing a membrane of division of self from self in the moment.

On this reading, concentric space as rapture offers a renewal of desiccated experience, not only of a dry brain in a dry season but for a dry experience in the stale air of the closure of diametric space; the fevered lip of the soft boundaries of concentric space renders a potential opening for experience beyond the sealed compartment of diametric spatial structures to engage with a greater dynamism and fluidity for experiential interaction with stimuli.

Concentric spatial experience offers a cessation of selfconsciousness where the self is an object of consciousness in diametric spatial terms of distanciation. This cessation of selfconsciousness may bring an acceleration of bliss, a dizzy rapture as a rush of fluidity prior to cognition. The emptying calls forth the concentric spatial relation as a possibility, although far from being an inevitability for experience. Concentric space is not being proposed as a nonsensory mode of experience, but as an accelerated expansion of the sensory through experience of the breath, as discussed in Downes (2012).

It is to be emphasised that concentric spatial projections underpinning experience are a structure of experience framing an infinite multiplicity of possible experiential contents as manifestations of concentric spaces' animating background; in similar vein, Nietzsche's Dionysian music is not to be reduced to one or a limited set of tunes. Concentric space is not to be reduced to a few repeated cognitions, attitudes or worldviews; it is much more dynamic than this and operates at a preconceptual, precognitive, prerepresentational framing level. As moisture for an experience prior to its compression or condensation into thought, it is not a prescription or description of particular cognitive constructs that are seeped into linear historical time.

Referring to women dancing 'in a trancelike state' (1976: 219), Kerenyi highlights that Dionysian enchantment was not simply one of wine-based intoxication (although centrally that), but also an enchantment akin to intoxication, as a deseating of the selfconscious observing mind.[14] Concentric spatial structures of relation are not to be equated with a one-to-one correspondence with any one specific mode of enchantment or ecstasy, as a dynamic movement of spatial projection. Rather it is a *spatial precondition* for such modes.

Concentric expansion of boundaries towards a heightened stimulation with background, towards an opening for background stimuli to invade awareness, nevertheless retains a sense of self as prereflective identity, the outer circle does not submerge the inner concentric circle. Concentric space retains a distinction between its poles, although one of common connection. Concentric space, unlike intoxication, does not *split* from self. In other words, while intoxication shares some features with concentric structured experience, as an unseating of selfconsciousness and accelerated opening of stimuli, intoxication does not sustain the subtlety of concentric structured experience. Concentric spatial awareness allows for a different kind of inwardness than a diametric split between inner and outer, it is not the reactive inwardness to instinctual energies being blocked that Nietzsche describes in GM.

Whether this unity described by Nietzsche is merely a fusion as a monism is open to question. While it is clear that Nietzsche struggles to accommodate the feature of concentric space as a relation of assumed connection for experience (such as his inability to encompass this for compassion), nevertheless, the relative openness and expansion of boundaries in concentric as distinct from diametric space, does run closer to Nietzsche's concerns, at least in his embracing of the Schopenhauerian *principium individuationis*. Yet even here, Nietzsche's framing of an expansion, an openness, is in terms of breaking and bursting open, of annihilating boundaries that is not a more fluid concentric movement.

The opening of the *principium individuationis* could be described as a concentric earthquake rippling through experience, yet it is notable that Kerenyi rejects any association between Dionysus and an eruptive experience: 'In all modern accounts of the Dionysian, an explosive trait has remained dominant. This is Nietzsche's dubious contribution' (1976: 138). This is a further gloss on the Dionysian by Nietzsche, an existential and phenomenological appendage to the historical factual descriptions of the Dionysian in ancient Greek times. Again this projection of emotional excess on the Dionysian by Nietzsche is revealing as a phenomenological account of an experiential process of opening or bursting open. Uncovering a concentric layer of experience may be a sudden bursting open or a more gradual flowing process.

Whereas intoxication risks annihilation of the diametric spatial boundaries and a lack of experiential fluidity and flexibility to return to an everyday boundaried state, a concentric spatial opening retains this fluidity afterwards and avoids a quasi-catatonic withdrawal into the monistic sealed world. The concentric may well be a bursting open from diametric to concentric structured experience, an *ekstasis* as expansion.

Concentric space is not a nostalgia for home, as a kind of romantic *Sehnsucht*; it is not a past-focused mode of experience. Neither is it a search for fixed, pregiven 'fragments of a secret treasure' (2000: 119), as Berlin describes the Enlightenment assumptions being challenged through romanticism; the fragments of concentric and diametric spaces are experiences to be felt and lived as part of a dynamism to generate system change, however, they are not pre-set, without the mediation of human experience, as a lived contextual content to animate the prior spatial-structural relations.

Both Nietzsche's Dionysian music and concentric structured experience offer a challenge to the Hegelian tenet of selfconsciousness as the essence of spirit. Moreover, it is to be emphasised that these spatial structures framing experience and thought are not being treated as selfconsciously present as images in thought; concentric space of assumed connection resists a subject–object distanciation that would place the image as an object of perception or thought, as a dimension of intentionality. These are proposed pre-intentional spaces of relation, shaping lived experience but not as simple selfconscious contents of experience.

This emphasis on a prior primordial spatial discourse is a challenge to a view of the unmediated will to life as shapeless chaos; Nietzsche is at the very least offering a monism as a spatial presupposition, and arguably more, for this experiential unity in a language prior to language that he envisages music as proffering. Spatialisation of thought exists whether Nietzsche likes it or not. His own language and conceptualisation, even of pre-image-based experience, is itself irredeemably spatial – and as argued in Chapter 9, this spatialisation is not merely reducible to metaphor, whether linguistic or conceptual metaphor. Spatialisation rather resides at a prior level of description with impact on subsequent levels and subsystems. It is to be emphasised that this prior spatial discourse is not a privileging of the visual modality; while it embraces all the senses, it is most strongly associated with experience of the breath prior to the senses (Downes 2012).

Nietzsche is emphasising the significance of a phenomenological shift from the Apollonian mode of experience, both for aesthetic experience and as conducive to a life principle. This phenomenological shift, at least in early Nietzsche, is not simply towards the aesthetic as simply the sensuous, as Heidegger characterises, focusing mainly on Nietzsche's *Nachlass*. A prior mediating spatial realm of experience is being invoked by the Nietzsche of BT, one not confined to the Procrustean ordering structure of the sensuous–nonsensuous opposition. While the Dionysian opening in experience may include a bodily component, it is primarily a primordial spatial opening, prior to a mind–body, nonsensuous–sensuous diametric opposition. Its radical restructuring is one that opens up beyond the very mode of diametric space itself. The gleams of half-extinguished concentric spatial possibilities haunt early Nietzschean rapture.

Critique of Heidegger's interpretation of Nietzsche's rapture

This spatial-phenomenological interpretation of Nietzsche's rapture does not rely on Schopenhauer's interpretation of Kantian aesthetics that Heidegger highlights is a misinterpretation; neither does it rest on Nietzsche's reaction to Schopenhauer that Heidegger treats as an inversion of Schopenhauer's already flawed interpretation. Heidegger argues (Vol. I: 108) that Schopenhauer misunderstood Kant's conception of the beautiful in *The Critique of Judgment* with regard to the phrase sheer delight 'devoid of all interest'. Schopenhauer treated this as apathy and disinterest, whereas Nietzsche responded to this through reversal as rapture. As Heidegger emphasises, Kant's phrase regarding interest, was to seek beauty as an end of itself, as a 'radiance ... coming to the fore' (Vol. I: 110), without being subservient to instrumental terms such as goals, intentions or individual advantages.

Yet this does not mean that Nietzsche's conception of rapture is thus 'misconceived' (Vol. I: 108), as Heidegger suggests. Heidegger neglects to give emphasis to the key phenomenological dimension of Schopenhauer's *principium individuationis*, accentuated by Nietzsche. Excision of this dimension from Nietzschean rapture, additional to the well-recognised minimising of the Dionysian elements to Nietzsche's thought in Heidegger (see, for example, Krell 1991) paves the way for Heidegger to treat Kant as a dominant reference point for Nietzsche via Schopenhauer. However, it is Schopenhauer's phenomenological account of the *principium individuationis* that offers major resonance with Nietzsche's own concerns and experiences.

Rather than treating Nietzsche's position as fundamentally derivative regarding rapture, as a reaction to a misunderstanding of Kant by Nietzsche via Schopenhauer, it needs to be understood, first, as a positive phenomenon on its own terms, as an insight building on Nietzsche's own experiences, as an experiential projection. And as such, Schopenhauer offers an edifice for Nietzsche's projection rather than being a direct source that would treat Nietzsche's insight as simply derivative from Schopenhauer. This is what Heidegger does more generally in choosing to relegate BT as one of Nietzsche's more minor works before his later insights regarding will to power (see Vol. I: 102–103) where he is viewed as coming into his own as an independent thinker.[15]

Rapture is being considered for current purposes quite apart from the question of its relation to the beautiful. Rather it is being interrogated as a life-giving process. Heidegger displaces focus from Schopenhauer's *principium individuationis* and early Nietzsche's reliance on it for understanding rapture, while nevertheless, retaining the centrality of rapture for Nietzsche's thought. Heidegger asks if rapture is a precondition for art but not if overcoming the *principium individuationis* is a precondition for rapture.

Heidegger interprets Nietzsche's rapture along an axis of sedative versus stimulant, as a reversal of Schopenhauer. Moreover, Heidegger imports a peripheral dimension to Nietzsche's concerns regarding rapture, namely Kantian beauty via an inversion of Schopenhauer, bringing this dimension of Schopenhauer to the forefront of his analysis. Heidegger accentuates this peripheral dimension to Nietzschean rapture, all the while that he largely neglects core features of Nietzsche's rapture – the Dionysian dimension and the *principium individuationis*; in contrast, the axis of openness versus closure, pivotal to the *principium individuationis*, is the key concern of Nietzsche with rapture.

Heidegger's shift away from Schopenhauer's *principium individuationis*, while privileging a Kantian centre of gravity for the analysis of aesthetic experience as rapture in Nietzsche, brings at least two implications. First, it moves away from an interpretation of rapture *in spatial terms.* [16] Second, it ignores and obscures the point that Nietzsche's rapture is in basic agreement here with Schopenhauer's account of challenge to the *principium individuationis*, rather than simply being an inversion of Schopenhauer's position (quite apart from further critique of metaphysical assumptions in a Schopenhauerean will). Schopenhauer and Nietzsche share a mutual concern with challenge to closure as an experiential mode of relation, they call into question the experiential retreat as expressed through the *principium individuationis.* [17] Their joint preoccupation is with overcoming a retreat into an inner citadel of diametric spatial closure.

While Heidegger acknowledges a Nietzschean concern with rapture as a life dimension, where 'life is life-enhancement and ascendant life is rapture' (Vol. I: 121), it is apparent that Heidegger locates rapture fundamentally in terms of later Nietzsche's will to power. However, as will to power is not to be simply blithely equated with life, but as a turning of and within a life principle (see Chapter 6), this brings a change to rapture as life and as a life-giving movement, in its reduction to serve power.

It can be argued that Heidegger at least implicitly invokes a concern with going beyond a mode of *principium individuationis*, when describing 'the essence of rapture and of beauty, namely ascent beyond oneself' (Vol. I: 116). This invites the question as to what is or is not the boundaries of oneself. Moreover, it fudges the issue of the kind of ascent, as an obliteration of boundaries invoking a fusion or as a concentric mode of expansion as assumed connection. The very image of ascent, with a higher/lower notion, while resonant with later Nietzsche's superman and self-surpassing, is not firmly focused on the axis of opening versus closure that the Schopenhauerean *principium individuationis* implicates.

Notably, Heidegger goes on to treat rapture as an explosion: 'Rapture as a state of feeling explodes the very subjectivity of the subject' (Vol. I: 123). Here Heidegger offers little beyond the view of the experiential state or form of rapture as annihilation of subjectivity. Heidegger views rapture as 'a unity of embodying attunement', with a 'feeling of plenitude' where 'nothing is foreign to it, nothing too much for it, which is open to everything and ready to tackle everything' (Vol. I: 100). This is a conception of rapture as an experiential process of inclusion of the other, through an absolutist openness, an openness to everything, consistent with obliteration of all boundaries. This is to be distinguished from a concentric spatial openness as *relative expansion.* Elsewhere Heidegger does describe Nietzschean rapture as 'the capacity to extend beyond oneself' (Vol. I: 100), which implies retention of self in this process, although without offering further structural exposition.

Heidegger emphasises Nietzsche's aesthetics as a physiology of art (Vol. I: 96), a rapturous feeling as a bodily state (Vol. I: 98). In doing so, it is Heidegger not Nietzsche that is trapped here in the sensuous/nonsensuous metaphysical opposition. The proposed spatial-phenomenological account of rapture treats it as a spatial experience prior to the sensory, but also offering bodily impacts and manifestations, although it is not confined to physiology or simple feeling. This is a spatial questioning of an opening for experience, building on Schopenhauer's *principium individuationis* and borrowed by Nietzsche who sought to invigorate it with a Dionysian gloss, a gloss not so much peeled away by Heidegger's analysis of rapture, as largely rendered invisible.

Conclusion

There is a need to distinguish openness as monism, as obliteration of self, and a concentric embedded bridging space, not above or beyond, but immersed in the background (ocean) as a mediating space. Put more metaphorically in Schopenhauerian terms, concentric space serves as a mediating space with the swirling storms, a wrapping principle as a surrounding mode of connective space to enable a swimming and not drowning in the ocean – as a healing and ecstatic space expanding through the primordial wound of life in the experiential abyss between foreground and background structures of experience.

It appears that for Nietzsche, like for many seminal thinkers, his life experiences ran ahead of the language and concepts within which he sought to house them; the accelerated movement into a realm of experience of the imageless that unseats the everyday boundaries of the individual swept past Nietzsche to a degree that he struggled to encapsulate this experience beyond a fiction in Dionysian terms and a pre-existing scheme of Schopenhauer's *principium individuationis*. Whereas early Nietzschean accounts of aesthetic experience as an elevated state of unity were wrapped in Dionysian apparel and further painted with a projective gloss of excess based on Nietzsche's own personal experience, a prior axis of a spatial protolanguage exists for this experiential terrain – a protolanguage invoking a monism as fusion and obliteration of self, concentric space as relative openness and connection, and diametric space as closure and assumed separation as a precondition for the subject–object division in everyday experience that is required to be subverted in aesthetic terms.

Key features of rapture are an opening as a restructuring of experience, as a prerepresentational mode of experience involving connection to an acceleration of stimuli as a rush, as a loss of boundaries of diametric spatial divisions between self and Other, self and environment, subject and object. This opening may lead to a loss of self as obliteration, as total fusion with externality, as explosion. The opening as a rush in experience brings a heightened awareness in the moment (with later echoes of Nietzsche's preoccupation with eternal recurrence in the moment). Awakening from the slumber induced by diametric spatial boundaries for experience brings an openness to the present moment. On this spatial-phenomenological reading, none of these features of rapture is associated with Dionysian features of ritual and repetition, of public festivals, of violence and sacrifice, or compensatory killing, as openness brings a heightened mode of connection rather than splitting. The question arises as to whether such an understanding of rapture needs to be tethered at all to the Dionysian edifice constructed by Nietzsche with scant recourse to historical fact and as a shell to house his experiential projections that may distract from its fundamental spatial structural dimensions for an experiential opening.

Concentric spatial features of Nietzche's rapture include a restructuring movement towards an opening, a shift from diametric spatial boundaries of splitting and assumed separation, immersion in a mode of prerepresentational experience based on an assumed connection prior to the distanciation of the subject–object division. This spatial opening for experience is not merely reducible to the physiological, although it may also have physiological manifestations. However, ultimately this opening is largely conceived by Nietzsche in monistic terms as fusion with background and obliteration of self (similar to Heidegger's interpretation of Nietzschean rapture as explosion), rather than as an accelerated mode of assumed connection with background in concentric space that allows for a dimension of self to be sustained in the experiential embedding with the rush of background stimuli.

The looser experiential boundaries of concentric structured experience in relation to the background stimuli allows for an openness that is resonant with a sense of enchantment or at least re-enchantment with the natural world. As direct lived experience, it is a mode of connective enchantment that is loosened from traditional conditioning processes with regard to the world, whether religious or secular conditioning patterns. Its first principles are experiential, seeped into the web of concentric structured experience, the bubble of connection as a transformation of everyday awareness, such as in awareness of breathing.

In the loosening of the diametric spatial boundaries there imports an apprehension of the moment, more intense, where experience is not simply a receptacle for stimuli but is one that dynamically interacts with stimuli in a moment of creation beyond mere reproduction of experience of the world. This is less so Dionysian rapture as the rapture of concentric space, the scent of which is sensed by Nietzsche but with a sense that is consistently bereft of both a connective mode and a dimension of self to be sustained in the momentary prereflective creation.

A life expanding concentric structured mode of more open experiential boundaries is possibly apprehended by Nietzsche through music as a pre-imagistic experience of the Dionysian. Nietzsche does offer concentric spatial imagery to describe the relation with music as the will in itself of life, 'the womb of the original unity' (BT: 119) 'the womb of music' (BT: 69). Against this backdrop, it can be concluded that even the 'freedom for' vision of music as unmediated will to life, despite some concentric imagery at the level of language and the appeal to a mode of prerepresentational experience prior to diametric spatial divisions needed for a subject–object dualism, is not predominantly a concentric spatial vision or plea for movement; it is rather a monism, an obliteration of boundaries. This view is also consistent with the characterisation of the Dionysian in Kerenyi as nature overpowering the mind. Consideration of Nietzsche's accounts of Dionysian intoxication leave little but the sense that this is a monistic fusion with an ocean, a will to life. The mind is overpowered in this process of surrendering individual identity, as part of an impersonal ecstasy. These are the contours of the unripe fruits of concentric space in early Nietzschean rapture.

Notes

1 Nietzsche subsequently retracts this position in his later work, rejecting BT's view of music as will in itself, unmediated, 'No music is in itself deep and full of meaning. It does not speak of the "will" or the "thing in itself" (HH: 128).
2 A continuity of concerns between BT's background ocean and storm together with the vessel of the *principium individuationis* can be found in later works of Nietzsche referring to the open sea and ships of GS, identifying the 'dark sea' with 'existence' (GS: 123), the ocean with 'the horizon of the infinite' (GS: 180) and Zarathustra's identification of selfovercoming with the ocean.
3 Kerenyi observes a strong interconnection between the Dionysian and Apollonian, treating them as not being mutually exclusive and even indistinguishable prophetically. He describes the Dionysian as the soil for Apollo, invoking a complementarity that appears also in places for Nietzsche in BT. However, Kerenyi (1976) explicitly takes Nietzsche to task for ignoring Dionysian women, for claiming all intoxication as Dionysian, for his dubious characterisation of the Dionysian as eruptive, while rejecting collective hysteria and Nietzsche's view of Dionysus as the hero of Greek tragedy.
4 See Downes (2012) on the illusory *samsara* in Buddhist thought in relation to diametric and concentric space.
5 Kant's noumenal/phenomenal contrasts are not part of this tradition, although central to Schopenhauer's account, as the noumenal is for Kant outside experience, unlike Schopenhauer's will in itself. An argument can be made that this foreground–background interaction is rooted in Plato's cave allegory, although Schopenhauer's emphasis is less reliant predominantly on the visual and embraces a wider phenomenological concern with the experiential and structures of the experiential; it is not the shadow on the cave and its source that is a Schopenhauerean concern, it is the experiential capacity to experience the shadow and experience beyond the shadow. Another in a Western tradition of foreground–background interaction is William James' (1890) stream of consciousness.
6 As Wagner notes with regard to this image of closure and loss of opening: 'Years later this image would give her the title of the novel … examining the stasis that made her feel that no matter what she did, "I would be sitting under the same glass bell jar, stewing in my own sour air"'(2000: 39).
7 Schopenhauer also anticipated the *Angst* of the existentialist movement with recognition of 'that indelible dread', 'an utterly dark presentiment' (WWRI: 379).
8 See also *satori* in Eastern traditions as imageless experience.
9 In similar vein to Davey, Ivanov views the Dionysian ecstasy is an 'ecstasy of impersonal happiness' springing from '*Taedium sui*, tiredness of one's particular individuality, freedom from the constraint of individual consciousness, from the prison of the ego' (quoted and translated in West 1970: 78) . Again on this existential interpretation, the Dionysian at least in Nietzsche's construction of tragedy is a response to a search for existential meaning.

10 'The hermeneutic significance of his stance is that it strives not to allow us to see the Greek world through Greek eyes, i.e., to reconstruct it in its own terms, but to look at our world through the tragic perspective of ancient Greece. That the radicality of Nietzsche's hermeneutic procedure has not been recognized or given its proper place within the history of modern hermeneutics is astonishing' Davey (1991: 112). For Davey, Nietzsche's 'approach to aesthetics is functionalist and genealogical from the start' (1991: 114).

11 For Bataille, 'not a word of Nietzsche's work can be understood without *experiencing* that dazzling dissolution into totality, without living it out' (1945: xxviii) recognising that lived experience is a fundamental concern. Bataille suggests that 'people do not believe in elevated states of soul, unless momentarily or at best over short periods of time – making exception for those few individuals who from experience know these elevated feelings in duration' (1945: 89). For Bataille: 'The tragedy of Nietzsche is the tragedy of night emerging from excesses of light' (1945: 101), so that an experiential fluidity is needed as a space to harness these excesses of light, as an opening that is not an obliteration.

12 It is to be recognised that Nietzsche's relation generally to romanticism is complex. As Parkes highlights: 'Nietzsche's criticisms in this period [just prior to BT] of the hypertrophy of cool, conscious rationality (soon to be associated with the figure of Socrates), as opposed to the deep, dark wellsprings of the creative unconscious, are very much in line with late Romanticist thinking about the creative process' (1994: 61). In contrast, as part of his argument to challenge affinities between Nietzsche and romanticism, Kaufmann (1975: 321) observes that Schlegel directly contrasted the classical *System des Kreislaufes*, which conceives history 'as a movement that returns upon itself in repeated cycles', with the modern romantic system of infinite progress (*System der unendlichen Fortschreitung*) (212). Kaufmann equates Goethe's view of romanticism as egoism coupled with weakness as 'the very essence of Nietzsche's conception of romanticism' (1975: 380). However, Kaufmann's emphasis that Nietzsche's later portrayal of the Dionysian changes into one 'associated with this very power of integration and self-discipline' (1975: 153), where the Dionysian is contrasted with the romantic and not the Apollonian is arguably a reconstruction of Nietzsche that goes a step too far.

13 Fitch observes that: 'Darwin's theory of musical protolanguage has had an oddly persistent tendency to be dissociated from its author's name, and to be rediscovered by later scholars. Many post-nineteenth-century champions of musical models fail to give proper acknowledgment to Darwin, even if they reference Darwin (1871) in some other connection (e.g. sexual selection ...)' (2010: 481). The question arises as to whether Nietzsche also falls into this category, albeit in the nineteenth century itself. With Darwin's hypothesis written in the year directly preceding BT, the question arises whether Nietzsche's appeal to a universal language of music was also influenced by Darwin's work, while recognising that elsewhere, such as in WP, Nietzsche sought to distance his positions from that of Darwinism.

14 Kerenyi notes: 'It is Homer who – in one of his rare mentions of the god – calls him *mainomenos* Dionysus, "mad Dionysus" ... Plato cites Homer and is for us his best interpreter. Women did not need wine when Dionysus intoxicated them: but their Dionysian intoxication seemed comparable to drunkenness' (1976:131). Thus, this intoxication is not the same as wine drinking but a shift from selfconsciousness to a more immediate awareness level.

15 Heidegger relegates the *principium individuationis* dimension through his relegation of BT, 'only in the years 1880 to 1883 did Nietzsche ... find himself as a thinker' (Vol. I: 8). Part of Heidegger's relegation of the importance of BT (see also Vol. I: 103 for his dismissive view of Nietzsche's Apollo/Dionysus opposition) is due to his view

that Hölderlin had identified the Apollo/Dionysus opposition in 'an even more profound and lofty manner' (Vol. I: 103). It is noteworthy that while Heidegger tends to minimise the importance of early Nietzsche's work such as BT, he nevertheless attributes extreme significance to the 19-year-old Nietzsche's insight regarding the eternal ring, as a precursor of eternal recurrence.

16 Heidegger does state: 'Form defines and demarcates for the first time the realm in which the state of waxing force and plenitude of being comes to fulfilment. Form founds the realm in which rapture as such becomes possible' (Vol. I: 119). This passage is amenable to interpretation in terms of concentric spatial structures, as a realm of opening for rapture, so that Heidegger's displacement from *principium individuationis* in spatial terms is not a deliberate excision of a fundamental spatial questioning, although a consequence of removing emphasis from this passage given centrality in early Nietzsche.

17 It is debatable whether the violence Heidegger seeks to do to Nietzsche's text regarding rapture, in the shift of attention from openness versus closure of Schopenhauer and Nietzsche's shared concern with the *principium individuationis* is any greater a violence than the 'misinterpretation' (Vol. I: 107) Heidegger attributes to Schopenhauer regarding his interpretation of Kantian beauty in terms of disinterest; Schopenhauer is arguably doing violence to Kant's text to turn apprehension of beauty into a mode more resonant with Eastern traditions of asceticism.

References

Bataille, G., *On Nietzsche*. Trans B. Boone. London/New York: Continuum, 1945/2004.

Berlin, I., *The Roots of Romanticism: The A. W. Mellon Lectures in the Fine Arts, 1965. The National Gallery of Art, Washington, DC*. H. Hardy (ed.). London: Pimlico, 2000.

Copleston, F., *Friedrich Nietzsche: Philosopher of Culture*. New York: Barnes & Noble Books, 1942/1975.

D'Aquili, E., 'The Influence of Jung on the Work of Claude Lévi-Strauss', *Journal of the History of the Behavioral Sciences*, 1975, 11: 41–48.

Davey, N., 'Hermeneutics and Nietzsche's Early Thought', in K. Ansell-Pearson (ed.), *Nietzsche and Modern German Thought*. London: Routledge, 1991, 88–118.

Descartes, R., *Descartes: Philosophical Writings* Trans. E. Anscombe and P.T. Geach. London: Nelson, 1954.

Downes, P., 'Cross-Cultural Structures of Concentric and Diametric Dualism in Lévi-Strauss' Structural Anthropology: Structures of Relation Underlying the Self and Ego Relation?', *Journal of Analytical Psychology*, 2003,48: 47–81.

Downes, P., *The Primordial Dance: Diametric and Concentric Spaces in the Unconscious World*. Oxford/Bern: Peter Lang, 2012.

Fitch, W. T., *The Evolution of Language*. Cambridge: Cambridge University Press, 2010.

Fodor, J. A., *The Language of Thought*. Hassocks: Harvester Press, 1976.

Frankopan, P., *The Silk Roads: A New History of the World*. London: Bloomsbury, 2015.

Freud, S., *The Interpretation of Dreams*. SE 4. London: Hogarth Press, 1900.

Freud, S., *Beyond the Pleasure Principle*. SE 18. London: Hogarth Press, 1920.

Fromm, E., *The Fear of Freedom*. London: Routledge, 1942.

Garfinkel, H., *Studies in Ethnomethodology*. Englewood Cliffs, NJ: Prentice Hall, 1967.

Heidegger, M., *Nietzsche*, Vols I and II. D. F. Krell (ed.), trans. D. F. Krell,. New York: HarperCollins, 1991.

Heidegger, M., 'Wilhelm Dilthey's Research and the Current Struggle for a World-view', in T. Kisiel and T. Sheehan (eds.), *Becoming Heidegger: On the Trail of his Early Occasional Writings 1910–1927*, 2nd revised, expanded ed. Seattle, Noesis Press, 2009.

Hofstadter, D. R., *Godel, Escher, Bach: An Eternal Golden Braid.* New York: Basic Books, 1979.

Hofstadter, D., *Metamagical Themas: Quests for the Essence of Mind and Pattern.* New York: Basic Books, 1985.

James, W., *The Principles of Psychology.* New York: Holt, 1890.

Kaufmann, W., *Nietzsche: Philosopher, Psychologist, Antichrist*, 4th ed. Princeton, NJ: Princeton University Press, 1975.

Kerenyi, C. *Dionysus: Archetypal Image of Indestructible Life.* Princeton, NJ: Princeton University Press, 1976.

Körner, S., 'The Impossibility of Transcendental Deductions', *Monist*, 1967, 51: 317–331.

Krell, D. F., 'Introduction to the Paperback Edition', in M. Heidegger, *Nietzsche*, Vols I and II. D. F. Krell (ed.), trans. D. F. Krell. New York: HarperCollins, 1991, ix–xxvii.

Lévi-Strauss, C., *The Savage Mind.* Trans. G. Weidenfeld, Nicolson Ltd. Chicago, IL: Chicago University Press, 1962.

Lévi-Strauss, C., *Structural Anthropology*, Vol. 1. Trans. C. Jacobsen and B. Grundfest Schoepf. London: Penguin, 1963.

Lévi-Strauss, C., *The Elementary Structures of Kinship.* Boston, MA: Beacon Press, 1969.

Lévi-Strauss, C., *The Raw and the Cooked: Introduction to a Science of Mythology* I. London: Jonathan Cape, 1970.

Lévi-Strauss, C., *Structural Anthropology*, Vol. 2. Trans. M. Layton. London: Penguin Books, 1973/1977.

Parkes, G., *Composing the Soul: Reaches of Nietzsche's Psychology.* Chicago, IL, University of Chicago Press, 1994.

Saussure, de F., 'NotesInédites de F.de Saussure', *Cahiers Ferdinand de Saussure*, 1954, 12.

Stambaugh, J., *The Other Nietzsche.* New York: State University of New York Press, 1994.

Thomson, I. D., *Heidegger, Art and Modernity.* New York: Cambridge University Press, 2011.

Wagner, E., *Ariel's Gift. Ted Hughes, Sylvia Plath and the Story of Birthday Letters.* London: Faber & Faber, 2000.

West, J., *Russian Symbolism: A Study of Vyacheslav Ivanov and the Russian Symbolist Aesthetic.* London: Methuen, 1970.

Wittgenstein, L., *Philosophical Investigations.* Oxford: Blackwell, 1958.

Wittgenstein, L., *On Certainty*, Oxford: Blackwell, 1969

Chapter 5

The spatial background between Dionysian and Apollonian myths

A prior spatial protolanguage in Nietzsche's Dionysus–Apollo relation as an optic of life: diametric space as figure–ground contrasts and monism that lacks an inclusion principle

The question arises as to whether Nietzsche can sustain a concentric spatial discourse, with regard to the *interaction* between the Dionysian and Apollonian, as well as more generally as a mediating structure of relation to embrace inclusion of the Other, of the counterpole, in his thought. Can Nietzsche's conception of the relation between the Dionysian and Apollonian, purportedly expressing the innermost foundation of life, embrace a concentric spatial relation of inclusion towards the other pole? Such a concentric structured discourse of inclusion as assumed connection is a level prior to simply linguistic images that express concentric modes, such as the 'womb of unity' and 'echo'. This invites a questioning as to the range of background relations that Nietzsche envisages to comprehend the interplay between his two poles of Dionysus and Apollo. As Kaufmann recognises: 'Nietzsche, however, fails to explain the relation of these forces to each other' and 'whether both can perhaps be reduced to a more basic conception' (1975: 177).

These relations can be understood in primordial spatial terms as the following: Figure–ground as a variant of diametric space, monism, diametric spatial opposition *simpliciter*, concentric space and the void.

Figure–ground as a variant of diametric space

Nietzsche predominantly conceptualises the Apollo–Dionysus relation as a figure–ground relation where both are in assumed separation from the other, yet mutually defining the other's shape: 'the reconciliation of two adversaries, clearly defining the boundaries to be respected' (BT: 25). As 'adversaries', they are fundamentally in a diametric space of assumed separation, which is the starting point from which a 'reconciliation' arrives as a figure–ground relation of some interaction. This is not a transformational restructuring but a figure–ground relation, as Nietzsche expressly refers to 'boundaries' being 'respected'.

This figure–ground relation is 'a relationship of reciprocal stimulation and intensification' (BT: 33), which is to 'run in parallel with one another' 'coupled with one another' (BT: 19). A parallel coupling again is consistent with a figure–ground duality. They are in a relation of complementary reciprocity as being mutually self-defining

Yet each can exist without the other. Thus, they are in a real and not simply modal distinction (Franks 2005).[1] This is also possible with figure–ground relations as each can exist in shape and meaning without the other, although their reciprocal relation can add 'intensification' to their mutual meaning. The opening paragraph of BT compares the Apollonian and Dionysian to intercourse between the sexes for 'more energetic births' (BT: 1). The sexual imagery to describe the relation between both at the outset of BT is very much resonant with a figure–ground relation, as both can exist in shape and meaning without the other; again reciprocal stimulation and intensification in a sexual sense offers a mode of interaction that still relies on two distinct entities coming together, as in a figure–ground reciprocity.

Whether treated as diametric dualistic spatial relations *simpliciter* or as a figure–ground reciprocal duality, as a variant of a diametric space of assumed separation, Nietzsche at times treats this Apollo–Dionysus duality in *sequential* terms. The Apollonian is 'objectivation' and rendering 'concrete' the Dionysian state (BT: 51), 'condensed into images' (BT: 52). This complementarity as a condensed sequential relation is where Apollo follows from Dionysus and the Apollonian is the 'completion' of the Dionysian 'state' (BT: 50). Such a sequential view gains some support from Kerenyi's historical account: 'the simplest, most unmistakable evidence of this relationship [between Apollo and Dionysus], without which the oracle could not have functioned, is the sacrifice of a goat: a Dionysian act preceding the Apollonian rite' (BT: 233).

Monism

A monistic relation between Dionysus and Apollo would take place where one is subordinated to the other. Such a monistic reduction of the Dionysian to the Apollonian (or vice versa) would give expression to 'Nietzsche's monistic tendency' (Faber, HH, 1994: xviii), already evident in his account of a monistic fusion with the background ocean and storm in overcoming the *principium individuationis*. Elsewhere Nietzsche rejects opposites such as unegoistic–egoistic, pleasure–displeasure (EH: 42), typically as part of a monism reducing one pole to really being subsumed in the other.

For Nietzsche, not only can each of Apollo and Dionysus exist without the other, each can subordinate the other. This offers limited support for a monistic relation between them. Nietzsche observes that the Apollonian 'triumphed completely over' the Dionysian and 'subordinated it to its aims' (BT: 116). Moreover, he challenges 'the illusion that the Dionysian is really in the service of the Apollonian' (BT: 115), as a monism where the Apollonian incorporates an enfeebled Dionysian. The seeds of a will to power exist here, where 'the Apollonian tears us away from the Dionysian' (BT: 115) and 'the Apollonian power breaks out' (BT: 114).

This power interplay offers 'a fraternal bond' (BT: 117) as 'the Dionysian again achieves predominance'; predominance is not quite a monistic reduction of the Apollonian to the Dionysian, but more a diametric hierarchy of mirror image reversal where one is in power and the other rendered relatively powerless. *Monism is the extreme within a diametric spatial mirror image inverted hierarchy.* Monism can be construed as the limiting condition for diametric space as hierarchical subordination of one pole to the other, where a mirror image of reversal of power/powerless lies at the extreme as an overwhelming of the powerless pole by the hegemony of the dominant one. The seeds of a diametric spatial will to power between the Apollonian and Dionysian are arguably stronger than any tendency in Nietzsche to treat these in purely monistic terms where one can be subsumed within the other.[2] A pure monistic reduction of one pole to the other would negate Nietzsche's core argument in BT that both these counterpoles are the preeminent features of Greek tragedy as a lens on life.

Diametric spatial opposition simpliciter

At times, Nietzsche conceptualises the Apollo–Dionysus relation in simple diametric spatial terms of mutual oppositional exclusion, 'wherever the Dionysian broke through, the Apollonian was cancelled, absorbed and annihilated' (BT: 32), 'its opposite' (BT: 23). This diametric spatial relation between Apollo and Dionysus is a construct of Nietzsche and is challenged at least in historical terms with regard to some dimensions by Kerenyi: '[I]n the prophetic realm Apollo and Dionysus are scarcely distinguishable' (1976: 219), 'the cult of Apollo ... by no means excludes a cult of Dionysus' (1976: 150). Similarly, West summarising Ivanov states:

> Apollo, mythologically speaking, only managed to hold his own in the conflict by usurping several Dionysian characteristics – the myths of Apollo and Dionysus became thoroughly intertwined, and eventually both gods were represented in the temple at Delphi. (1970: 80)

Nevertheless, Nietzsche's tendency to place the Apollonian and Dionysian in diametric spatial opposition is not without some historical support, as evinced by Kerenyi, as Dionysus is 'the dark god' and Apollo 'the luminous god' (1976: 233), thereby envisaging a mirror image relation of inversion between both. The key issue once again for current purposes is less historical accuracy of the Dionysian in Nietzsche but rather the emotional excess, the projected structures of relation underpinning his thought in general, and with regard to the Dionysian in its interplay with the Apollonian.

A further clear diametric spatial opposition in BT is the 'new opposition' between the Dionysian and the Socratic where 'the logical nature … developed itself to excess', and 'the logical drive' is identified with 'the Socratic way of life' (BT: 75) leading to a scenario where 'science annihilated myth' (BT: 93); Socrates epitomises for Nietzsche the 'abstract man' (BT: 122), leading to 'annihilation of myth' (BT: 123). Nietzsche treats the Socratic as an extremity within the Apollonian, 'the Apollonian tendency has disguised itself in logical schematism' (BT: 78) as a kind of sublimation of the Apollonian myth. The Socratic on this view is an extremity of the Apollonian in its counterpoint to the Dionysian.

Whereas aspects of the Dionysus–Apollo relation can be treated as a figure–ground relation of some reciprocal interaction, although based on assumed separation, as a variant of diametric opposition, the Dionysian–Socratic opposition is pure diametric spatial opposition. This view distinguishing figure–ground diametric spatial opposition from diametric spatial dualism *simpliciter* offers a basis for Smith's recognition that for Nietzsche in BT, the 'real enemy' (2000: xix) of Dionysus is not the Apollonian but the Socratic rationalism that comes to the fore in Euripides.[3]

A firm opposition of diametric space *simpliciter* as assumed separation in Nietzsche's later commentary on BT treats its 'decisive innovations' of BT (EH: 45) as not only 'understanding of the Dionysian phenomenon' (EH: 46) but also understanding of Socrates' rationality as 'a dangerous life-undermining power' (EH: 46). This again supports a view of a real enemy of pure diametric opposition as being that between the Dionysian and the Socratic, with the Dionysus–Apollo opposition being a figure–ground more moderate opposition, nevertheless resting on the basic assumption of separation between both poles, as a defining feature of diametric space.

Promissory notes towards a concentric spatial relation? A transformational relation short of dissolving

In some places, Nietzsche appears to offer a further integrated affinity, where he treats Apollo and Dionysus as 'interwoven' and in dialectical relation[4] leading to a further synthesis, so that the 'origin and essence of Greek tragedy, as the expression of two interwoven artistic drives' (BT: 68). This interweaving relation is consistent with a concentric spatial relation. Across BT, however, there is little sense of *containment* of the Apollonian in the Dionysian or vice versa, for a concentric spatial relation. One is not surrounded by the other through a major restructuring (or *encountered* in the Heideggerian sense; see Chapter 10).

Among the array of relations postulated between both poles in BT, it is difficult to locate any definitive example of a concentric relation of mutual transformation – in all the envisaged modes, the boundaries of each pole are either retained or annihilated, they are not restructured as such through a modification or transformation. Nietzsche seeks to 'dismantle stone by stone the elaborate edifice of Apollonian culture' (BT: 26). This is not a dissolving as a freshening through incorporation. Gain or growth of the Dionysian is *not through inclusion but through imposition – through imposing one on the other in order to simply negate or exclude the other.* Lévi-Strauss describes this crucial difference between *negation–imposition* and *dissolving* generally:

> [...] I believe the ultimate goal of the human sciences to be not to constitute, but to dissolve man ... I am not blind to the fact that the verb 'dissolve' does not in any way imply (but even excludes) the destruction of the constituents of the body subjected to the action of another body. The solution of a solid into a liquid alters the disposition of its molecules. It also often provides an efficacious method of putting them by so that they can be recovered in case of need and their properties be better studied. (1962: 247)

The dissolving changes not only the solid but also the fluid into which the solid is being dissolved; it is a two-way change process and needs to be distinguished from destruction as negation.

The question arises as to whether the following transformation could be construed as a dissolution, when Nietzsche suggests 'this dismemberment, the properly Dionysian suffering, is similar to a transformation into earth, wind, fire and water' (BT: 59). However, dismemberment is fundamentally a splitting process, a diametric spatial movement even when treated here as an elemental transformation as a kind of sublimation. It is not a question of razing to the ground a diametric space but rather of its incorporation into the concentric, as part of its dissolution as a restructuring. A transformative spatial movement rests outside Nietzschean horizons here.

Elsewhere, in Zarathustra, through which the Dionysian is pervasive, 'all opposites are fused together into a new unity' (EH: 72), 'containing within itself all opposites' (EH: 81). This offers a notion of containment. However, it is far from apparent that this is envisaged as a concentric spatial kind of containment, beyond the rhetorical term containment. Nietzsche is far from being explicit on their propensity to be engaged in a mutual transformational change as a dissolving process of the diametric into the concentric pole, of a radical integration that is not mere annihilation of the counterpole but its incorporation. Nietzsche treats dissolving as a mere annihilation rather than a concentric kind of restructuring, 'the abyss of annihilation must experience the dissolution of nature' (BT: 55); he does not distinguish dissolving and annihilating.

Heidegger places emphasis on Nietzsche's term 'incorporation' as 'the plan's key word' (Vol. II: 75), in the Four Notes dated August 1881 on eternal return. This includes 'incorporation of the passions'. As Heidegger highlights: 'If we pursue the meaning of the word we arrive at the notion of "eating", of devouring and digesting. Whatever is incorporated makes the body – and our embodiment – steadfast and secure' (Vol. II: 76). This conception of incorporation is close to dissolving as a transformation; dissolving is a material incorporation, although not necessarily limited to a bodily process. Incorporation also invites roots to Dionysian rituals, although this is not emphasised by Heidegger. Nevertheless, neither dissolving as an inclusion of the opposite counterpole nor incorporation as a more bodily restructuring bringing an integration into an assumed connection between the Dionysian and Apollonian are prevalent in BT.

Parkes appears to envisage a Dionysian–Apollonian relation that offers a mode tantamount to a concentric spatial relation building on Nietzsche's account in *Twilight of the Idols*, 'a Dionysian life that is no longer in opposition to Apollonian existence but has superseded it by incorporating and going beyond it' (1994: 358). Parkes extracts: 'The schema developed by Nietzsche – (1) natural anarchy [of drives] (2) disciplined self-tyranny, and (3) enlightened spontaneity' (1994: 459). Likewise, a concentric mode of inclusion of each dimension within a concentric spatial relation is a possible implication from the understanding of Ivanov. Apollo and Dionysus complete each other, according to Ivanov:

> Though Apollo may emerge from the struggle transformed, Dionysus too is made lighter and purer. It is a synthesis of the two deities that first sets the seal on the Greek idea ... Each god completes the other, as the golden vision of Apollo's charms quells the ecstatic turbulence of the musical intoxication. (Ivanov, quoted and translated in West 1970: 80)

This is not just a zero sum game, as in much of Nietzsche, but a mutually transforming synthesis.

The void

BT's interplay between the Apollonian and Dionysian is as a response to experience of an existential void. Davey observes 'a common existential predicament' (1991: 109), while accepting that 'Nietzsche clearly recognises that the Greek sense of existential nausea cannot be straightforwardly the same as that experienced by a post-Christian European' (1991: 107). Davey's position on the existentialist vantage point of Nietzsche is resonant with Nietzsche's accounts of 'a tremendous void [that] encircled man' (GM: 117), where asceticism is an existential response to the void where 'he suffered from the problem of his own meaning' (GM: 118).[5]

Heidegger's commentary on Nietzsche invokes the void (Vol. II: 89) as a dimension prior to space. Yet this very conception requires more contextualisation than as an abstract void, bereft of interaction with space. The void can be interpreted as the split background relation between diametric and concentric space, although this is more a diametric spatial splitting as a splitting invites at least the possibility of change to overcome this split; the void is better considered here as a nonrelation between concentric and diametric space, lacking even the potential for relation between them or change to this state. The void can also be construed as the collapse of diametric spatial structures. A diametric space offers a relation, albeit a limited one in terms of opposition and splitting; it holds opposites in at least a minimal relation. A further dimension of the void is as a failure to even establish an initial diametric or concentric spatial relation between dimensions or entities. The void as a non-space must thus still be considered spatially, in embedded contextual terms for experience, rather than as sheer abstraction; the void as a non-space still beckons a relation to fundamental spatial modes of relation. The void as a lack of capacity for space, not even as a potentiality or as a loss of space, can still be related to space as a discordance from space.

Heidegger cites Nietzsche on a conception of space that, 'first emerged by virtue of the supposition of an empty space. There is no such thing. All is force' (XII, no.98) and treats this as leading to the trail of 'the fundamental phenomenon of the void' which 'does not necessarily have to do merely with space, or with time either ... the essence of Being could include the void' (Vol. II: 89) – as strife. Surprisingly, Heidegger does not interpret Nietzsche's statement, at least not directly, in terms of its rejection of Cartesianism, of an empty space founding abstraction and cognitive modes of experience (see also Downes 2006, 2010, 2010a).

The domain of relevance for Nietzsche's rapture pertains to an experiential restructuring in specific spatial terms. These spatial terms conveyed metaphorically by Schopenhauer in his account of the *principium individuationis* as the frail vessel on the ocean can be examined as specific spatial-phenomenological structures of experience, namely, as diametric space *simpliciter*, figure–ground as a variant of diametric space, monism, concentric space and the void. These spaces may have a bodily impact but are not simply bodily. Heidegger's focus on aesthetics regarding Nietzsche's and Schopenhauer's misinterpretation of Kant on beauty is a sidetrack from this key insight of Schopenhauer, amplified by Nietzsche in BT, concerning the *principium individuationis*. It is surprising that Heidegger overlooked this experiential axis of opening and closure in Nietzschean rapture, as movement in the moment from the boundaries of the *principium individuationis* of Schopenhauer, given that eternal recurrence and its dimension of the moment accentuated by Heidegger is resonant with an opening in the moment through rapture. This is not the only central feature of Nietzsche's account of rapture radically minimised by Heidegger, the other being the Dionysian dimension to rapture constructed by Nietzsche. Interrogation of the Dionysus–Apollo relation in BT in spatial phenomenological terms invites a conclusion that their mutual relation is far from being a concentric spatial one of assumed connection as mutual overlapping qualities that resist fusion into monism, but is most consistently portrayed as a figure–ground variant of diametric space.

Nietzsche's dance between the Dionysian and Apollonian is on this spatial-phenomenological reading a derivative set of gestures from a prior, more fundamental primordial dance between concentric and diametric spaces of experience. Concentric and diametric spatial structures of experience coalesce with each other in a dance where each needs and beckons the other.

Hermeneutic approaches in a spatial-phenomenological reading of Nietzsche

Rather than on focusing on the Husserlian phenomenological tenet, 'to the things themselves', the angle of interrogation is *to the spaces themselves*, the mobile spaces in their dancing interplay. This spatial-phenomenology is a phenomenology *through* space rather than perception of objects or images *in* space (Downes 2012). This proposed framework of spatial-phenomenology seeks to lay bare how basic concepts that glue together human understanding are all irretrievably condemned to spatial claims, to resting on implicit or explicit spatial assumptions. These spatial preoccupations underpinning Nietzsche's thought can help understand Nietzsche as being not only a thinker resonant with existentialist traditions but also with phenomenological concerns with both lived experience and structures of experience; the leap is from Nietzsche's apprehension of patterns to interpretation of these patterns in spatial terms, and not only in terms of phenomenology but also a specific spatial-phenomenology of diametric and concentric spaces.

Nietzsche's problematizing of the true–false diametric opposition is as part of his ultimate quest to be free not only of the sensuous–supersensuous metaphysical opposition, but also of the attributions of truth and falsity, appearance and reality that governs this whole framework. In doing so, he placed the aesthetic before the true, as part of his reconstruction of these valuations. A different approach is taken for current purposes of a spatial-phenomenology. The proposed common set of spatial projections of modes of experience as chambers of space for understanding brings an added level of explanation beyond contrasts between foreground images and perceived objects in space and a background level of concepts and ideas; it offers a further background to the background, where concepts and ideas are wrapped in spatial assumptions. In doing so, it relativises the very conception of what is or is not foreground and background. Truth claims are relativised to the level of description in the network of foreground–background interactions, while even the terms foreground and background become relative to the level of description. Surveying these cavernous terrains of space for truth claims brings a relativity of interpretation, depending on vantage point; relativity is different *in toto* from a mere relativism of truth claims.

It might be objected that interpretation of the Dionysian in terms of concentric and diametric spaces is a quasi-Apollonian attempt to impose form on what Nietzsche treats as a formless expansive sea. However, it is not being sought to impose any such form but rather to uncover structural regularities in Nietzsche's own habits of thought and experience, his own silent background projections. These are being argued to exist as a prior spatial proto-language to the Dionysian–Apollonian opposition, whether or not one has a predilection or not for the Dionysian. Moreover, as structures of experience projected into concepts and language they are being treated *not as forms* split from experiential content but as *structures that are continuous with content* of experience (Downes 2010, 2012). Furthermore, emphasis on a spatialisation in Nietzsche's thought is consistent with a physicality, an embodiment that is a feature of Nietzsche's critique of mere abstraction and a metaphysical beyond. These spaces are being examined as already embedded into the fabric of Nietzsche's thought, as projections of his experience and of primordial experience.

A danger with reading Nietzsche is the selective citation of isolated passages that run in direct antithesis to other parts of his thought, as part of the maze of his contrary conceptual trajectories. This would bring simply a 'polymorphous' Nietzsche 'available to all camps' Pippin (1991: 283). Levels typically distinguished in Nietzsche's work and beyond this, are use of imagery and linguistic metaphor that may, for example, offer concentric imagery, as distinct from a conceptual level[6] in concentric structured terms. Parkes observes in Nietzsche:

> [A]n inner space of planets, moons, and galaxies; an 'inscape' of land and sea, rocks and waves, sun and winds. This notion of inner space is prefigured in other philosophers – in Saint Augustine especially … it is generally foreign to ancient Greek thinking, where the distinction between inner and outer was not well developed. (1994: 127)

Yet this focus is predominantly on objects *in* space rather than on the mode of the space itself, while also operating at the level of imagery more than conceptual structure.

In drawing out contrasts with Nietzsche, Parkes recognises these different linguistic and conceptual levels where Plato's imagery is frequently in tension with his thought: 'It is surprising that Plato should employ metaphors drawn from the vegetable or animal realms at all, in view of the way his metaphysics privileges the heavens and the realm of the intellect over the earth and the body' (1994: 172). A similar argument is being made here with regard to Nietzsche's imagery and thought, namely, that linguistic metaphor and conceptual assumptions lie in contrast with one another, not only as a cacophonous clash, but also as being illustrative of the need to distinguish these levels for spatial-phenomenological concerns. This selfreferential tension between the poetic and conceptual does not negate the relevance of either as levels of description. The possibility also exists that these levels may be in possible harmony as a selfreferential consistency, although this cannot be assumed to actually occur.

It is the conceptual structure of Nietzsche's basic concepts that is being interrogated in spatial terms, not especially his linguistic imagery, although with some exceptions such as for the imagistic understandings of eternal recurrence. The foreground–background distinction is a relative one, so that a background focus on spatial structures of relation is distinct from a foreground focus on imagery, on images in space or objects in space. It involves a scrutiny of assumptions of understanding, horizons of understanding relying on spatial assumptions.

It is very much recognised that there are other interesting ways of interpreting Nietzsche's works focusing particularly on his language, given his propensity for imagistic thinking, highlighted, for example, by Parkes' (1994) account of his imagery in terms of elements (earth, water, fire, air), vegetal and agricultural metaphor, as well as natural process images in terms of animals and human procreation. This imagery focused level brings not only a rich source of multiplicity for interpreting Nietzsche but also many fluid images that are resonant with concentric spaces at a linguistic level.

A counterargument to a distinction between analytical levels of Nietzsche's imagery and conceptual levels is that of Scheiffele who suggests that Nietzsche's 'form of thinking cannot be separated from the content' with 'a primary feature of Nietzsche's perspectivism: namely, *the "estranging" of what is one's own by questioning it from behind (hinterfragen), from the perspective of the foreign*' (1991: 32). However, examination of the diametric spatial structure in conceptual assumptions opens up and does not suppress a questioning of the foreign.

In similar vein, Heidegger's later work emphasises the key role of poetic thinking, and rejects a distinction between the poetic and theoretical, including for reading Nietzsche's work.[7] This is especially apt, for example, for consideration of Nietzsche's eternal recurrence, which is particularly expressed imagistically. However, the spatial-phenomenological concerns with background spatial structure is *not a space that derives from language as the poetic* but is argued to be prior to language. Nevertheless, this prior spatial level of questioning of the assumption structure of concepts does actively interact with language and foreground images, so the distinction is one that is on the basis of assumed connection between levels rather than a rigid bifurcation. It is a difference of emphasis and degree as an interpretative approach from one focusing on the multiplicity of Nietzsche's images and linguistic metaphors.

A necessary dialectical tension takes place between both hermeneutic approaches. This is not an argument that the spatial-phenomenological approach is a sole, monolithic approach to interpreting texts; its goal is not truth totality but a directional unity. It is to be recognised that this itself lies in tension with many readings of Nietzsche who disavows systematisation; a will to system is not being advocated but rather it is being argued that a system is already in operation in Nietzsche's conceptual assumptions, a silent system of disavowed space.

Parkes highlights that Nietzsche: 'traces apparent unities back to underlying multiplicities – a reversal, in a sense, of the movement of Platonic dialectic' (1994: 249), where: 'The most radical feature of Nietzsche's psychology – generally neglected or not well understood in the secondary literature – is his conception of the psyche as a multiplicity, in contrast with the traditional idea of the soul as something unitary' (1994: 251). This emphasis on multiplicities rather than unities for Nietzsche is apt at the level of imagery and linguistic metaphor, however, arguably less so at a conceptual or at least structural level. Much depends on the level of description for ascribing a priority of Nietzsche to multiplicity or unity, while recognising the need to challenge simple static unities.[8]

A Nietzschean concern with multiplicity operates most directly at the foreground level of description with regard to imagery and some conceptual aspects. However, at a background spatial-structural level different structural concerns gain vitality. Reconciliation of this position with Parkes' emphasis can take place with recognition of Nietzsche's concern with some kind of ordering within multiplicity, that it is not a mere chaos of multiple drives prior to the flawed unities Nietzsche perceives in Western traditions, such as the soul atomism of Christianity, the good–evil constructs of slave morality and the Cartesian ego. A background ordering principle exists in rudimentary form in Nietzsche's thought, a principle amenable to interpretation in spatial-structural terms, though as will be argued, these background spatial ordering principles are incomplete in Nietzsche's thought.

Parkes is 'highly suspicious of any programs' such as that of Schiller's proposing to subject (1994: 261) the multiplicity within to an ideal unity. This gains support from Nietzsche's rejection of a naive teleology as ideal form; Heidegger (Vol. II: 93) cites Nietzsche: 'Let us guard against believing that the universe displays a tendency to achieve certain forms, that it wants to become more beautiful, more perfect, more complex! All of that is humanization!' (XII, 111). Movement from diametric to concentric spatial systems is not an ideal unity as abstraction, locked with an ideal–real opposition. Neither is it some quasi-Hegelian inevitable march towards a preconceived teleological goal. It is rather a fragile directional spatial movement, as a potential structure of experience projected into understandings at the level of coherent implicit assumption structures governing seminal concepts.

Notes

1 This is expressed by Franks in the following terms: 'In the Cartesian tradition … X and Y are really distinct if each *can exist* when the other does not; X and Y are modally distinct if either one can exist when the other does not, but not vice-versa' (2005: 54f).

2 For Kaufmann, 'the assumption of a single basic principle' in later Nietzsche of will to power is treated as 'a reconciliation … finally effected between Dionysus and Apollo' (1975: 178). This is treated as a shift from dualism of his earlier

work to what develops into 'an all-embracing monism' (1975: 192), going beyond simply human experience, to the animal kingdom and to a wider cosmological principle.

3 However, Parkes observes Socrates' 'eminently realistic attitude towards the omnipresence of brutal desires'(1994: 225) so that Nietzsche's characterisation of Socrates as extolling sheer abstraction is an oversimplification of Socrates' position. Again, Parkes suggests that characterising Socrates as a tyranny of reason does not do justice to Socrates' position (1994: 351). Moreover, Kaufmann challenges the 'dogma' (1975: 391) that Nietzsche repudiated Socrates.

4 See also Kaufmann (1975:157).

5 For Nietzsche, it is: 'Not suffering, but the senselessness of suffering was the curse … the ascetic ideal gave it a meaning' (GM: 118). A response to suffering is his whole work and search for existential meaning. The ascetic can be construed as a desire for active control rather than being a passive recipient of suffering; it is a diametric mirror image spatial inversion strategy, resonant with the desire to be active highlighted as part of Freud's compulsion to repeat.

6 This is in the sense of the contrast between linguistic and conceptual metaphor offered by Lakoff and Johnson (1980). Similarly, Parkes distinguishes 'the track of Nietzsche's metaphorics … [with] a shift to the conceptual, involving an elaboration of ideas rather than images for the workings of the soul' (1994: 249).

7 For Heidegger: 'In Nietzsche's thinking of his fundamental thought the "poetical" is every bit as "theoretical" and the "theoretical" is inherently "poetical"' (Vol. II: 73).

8 As Parkes accentuates, 'a main trait of the genealogical method to take what appears to be a unitary phenomenon and disclose its multiple origins, showing it to be generated by a plurality of drives' (1994: 277). However, Parkes also recognises the other level of description for Nietzsche's conceptual assumption in terms of a monism, Nietzsche's will to power 'can be seen as the culmination of monistic tendencies in the tradition from Leibniz and Spinoza through the German Romantic thinkers as epitomized by Herder' (Parkes 1994: 316).

References

Davey, N., 'Hermeneutics and Nietzsche's Early Thought', In K. Ansell-Pearson (ed.), *Nietzsche and Modern German Thought*. London: Routledge, 1991, 88–118.

Downes, P., 'Newtonian Space: The "Blind Spot" in Newell and Simon's Information Processing Paradigm', *Cybernetics and Human Knowing*, 2006, 13: 25–55.

Downes, P., 'Schema Structure-Content Relativity: Part II, From Image Schemata to Background Spatial Schemata of Diametric and Concentric Relation', *Cybernetics and Human Knowing*, 2010, 17: 25–43.

Downes, P., '"Newtonian Space in Newell and Simon: Reply to Kinsella's (2008) response to Downes (2006)', *Cybernetics and Human Knowing*, 2010a,17(1): 191–200.

Downes, P., *The Primordial Dance: Diametric and Concentric Spaces in the Unconscious World*. Oxford/Bern: Peter Lang, 2012.

Faber, M., *Editor's Introduction to F. Nietzsche, 'Human All Too Human'*. London: Penguin, 1878.

Franks, P., *All or Nothing: Systematicity, Transcendental Arguments and Scepticism in German Idealism*. Cambridge, MA: Harvard University Press, 2005.

Heidegger, M., *Nietzsche*, Vols I and II. D. F. Krell (ed.), trans. D. F. Krell. New York: HarperCollins, 1991.

Hulin, M., 'Nietzsche and the Suffering of the Indian Ascetic', in G. Parkes (ed.), *Nietzsche and Asian Thought*. Trans. G. Parkes. Chicago, IL: University of Chicago Press, 1991.

Kaufmann, W., *Nietzsche: Philosopher, Psychologist, Antichrist*, 4th ed. Princeton, NJ: Princeton University Press, 1975.

Kerenyi, C., *Dionysus: Archetypal Image of Indestructible Life*. Princeton, NJ: Princeton University Press, 1976.

Lakoff, G. and Johnson, M., *Metaphors We Live By*. Chicago, IL: University of Chicago Press, 1980.

Lévi-Strauss, C., *The Savage Mind*. Trans. G. Weidenfeld, Nicolson Ltd. Chicago, IL: Chicago University Press, 1962/1966.

Martin, G. T., 'Deconstruction and Breakthrough in Nietzsche and Nagàrjuna', inG. Parkes (ed.), *Nietzsche and Asian Thought*. Trans. G Parkes. Chicago, IL: University of Chicago Press, 1991.

Parkes, G., *Composing the Soul: Reaches of Nietzsche's Psychology*. Chicago, IL: University of Chicago Press, 1994.

Pippin, R., 'Nietzsche, Heidegger and the Metaphysics of Modernity', In K. Ansell-Pearson (ed.), *Nietzsche and Modern German Thought*. London: Routledge, 1991, 282–310.

Scheiffele, E., 'Questioning One's "Own" from the Perspective of the Foreign by Eberhard Scheiffele', in G. Parkes (ed.), *Nietzsche and Asian Thought*. Trans. G. Parkes. Chicago, IL: University of Chicago Press, 1991.

Smith, D., *Introduction to Nietzsche's 'The Birth of Tragedy'*. Trans. D. Smith.

Oxford: Oxford University Press, 2000.

West, J., *Russian Symbolism: A Study of Vyacheslav Ivanov and the Russian Symbolist Aesthetic*. London: Methuen, 1970.

Chapter 6

Power and space

> 'Then, what is Life?'
>
> Shelley 'The Triumph of Life' (1822)

Nietzsche's will to power as a diametric spatial inversion of a life principle

Concentric space as a structure of inclusion appears to be anathema to at least the later Nietszschean extolling of the will to power: 'The will that is the will to power must will something higher than any reconciliation' (Z: 163). This is far from any conception of inclusion. Nietzsche's will to power rejects even the potential for inclusion as reconciliation, offering an entrenched habit of maximum distanciation. The will to power is not an integrative process of assumed connection, as a concentric spatial movement.

Nietzsche is far from being the first to relate life with power.[1] Shelley's *Mont Blanc*, for instance, describes: 'All things that move and breathe with toil and sound/Are born and die ... Power dwells apart in its tranquillity' with Mont Blanc epitomising power: 'Mont Blanc gleams on high: the Power is there' (1817/2002: 99–100). However, Nietzsche's conception of the relation between life and power is a subtle one, with multiple strands that go beyond treating life and power as being in a relation of simple equivalence or residing firmly apart. This relation requires clarification in spatial structural terms, especially of diametric space.

Without resiling from Nietzsche's celebration of multiplicity, it is being argued that Nietzsche repeatedly illustrates the operation of will to power in spatial-structural terms as diametric space, with regard to a) diametric spatial features of splitting and, most prominently, b) mirror image reversal including inversions as power hierarchy, and c) closure including repetitive rituals, seeped also into the very fabric of the Dionysian in ancient Greece.

Will to power as splitting through a diametric spatial movement

Nietzsche envisages an oppositional process within life itself: '[H]owever much I love it – soon I have to oppose it' (Z: 138); 'Spirit is the life that itself strikes into life: through its own torment it increases its own knowledge' (Z: 127). This striking, oppositional, dividing process is where life turns towards the goal of knowledge, with an association here of spirit with knowledge. Although not explicitly in diametric *spatial* terms, it is clearly construed by Nietzsche in diametric oppositional terms, which itself presupposes a spatial background manifestation.

A key preoccupation of Nietzsche is with that of hardness, cutting and dividing. This all feeds into diametric space as a dynamic process of assumed separation, as a movement of splitting. Nietzsche envisages this process as occurring in primordial terms: '[T]his eternal foundation upon hard primordial rock, upon this highest, hardest primordial hill' (Z: 253), 'the dividing place of storms' (Z: 254) where the ocean storms of the background to the *principium individuationis* have given way to diametric spaces as a dividing process, where 'spirit is the life that itself cuts into life' (Z: 264), 'with my own blood I have increased my knowledge' (Z: 264). He exhorts to 'become hard!' 'creators are hard' (Z: 231), '*all creators are hard*, is the true badge of a Dionysian nature' (EH: 76). Not only is the assumed separation movement of diametric space a splitting process associated with the primordial and the Dionysian, it is explicitly linked to destruction as an end of itself, including though going beyond an instrumental organic pruning process: 'For a Dionysian task the hardness of the hammer, *the pleasure even in destroying* are crucial preconditions' (EH: 76). Treating philosophy as a hammer, Nietzsche invokes a spirit as 'anvil ... hammer' (Z: 128). In doing so, he risks the accusation that having a hammer, he can only see an environment of nails, and he is nailed himself to the projective process of diametric space. With this engulfment in diametric spatial opposition, Nietzsche is swept along on the diametric movement of assumed separation as splitting, with 'the *joy of destruction*' (EH: 47), 'saying 'yes' to opposition and war' (EH: 48). Diametric space is Nietzsche's silent sword and scalpel.

A sword of diametric space eats into itself, cashing in its rust against its own ferocity. The rage of the diametric loses all-aroundness, where anger craves its crust. Later Nietzsche transports a background of original pain into a will to power, as a diametric space where Schopenhauer is treated as 'wrong about everything', as he rejects his earlier thought 'tainted with the doleful scent of Schopenhauer' (EH: 45) (including presumably being wrong about the will to life, not only as a will in itself claim). In some passages, later Nietzsche is tethered to a monism reducing soul to body and rejects '"pain in the soul" as a real fact' (GM: 93). Yet the fundamental shift here in Nietzsche is from an earlier mode of relative openness, of loosening and expansion of awareness to enter the storms of an original pain and its concentric echoes (ultimately devouring individual identity in a monistic fusion). Instead, he resorts to a mode of exertion of power on the storms of the original pain, so that the will to power inflicts suffering and is not simply a passive recipient of suffering.

Nietzsche's will to power offers a different response to the problem of the *principium individuationis*; rather than overcome the frail vessel of the boat to enter the ocean and swirling storms to become one with it as a fusion, the will to power seeks to bring division of diametric space, where storms become a 'dividing place' (Z: 254), as a domain for the exertion of power of the frail vessel. The vessel's role is subjected to a mirror image inversion of function, from a fragile closure to the overpowering storms to the later exertion of strength as power over the storms and to thereby divide them. The earlier response challenges a retreat into the *principium individuationis* of diametric space of the closed compartment of the frail vessel, the latter one is an aggressive expansion as imposition of a diametric space as a dividing structure to be imposed on the background storm.

This saturation of diametric spatial assumptions in later Nietzsche's thought is further manifested in his account of spirit. He portrays 'a fundamental will of the spirit' in will to power terms:

> That imperious something which is popularly called 'the spirit' wishes to be master internally and externally, and to feel itself master … a binding, taming, imperious and essentially ruling will … The power of the spirit to appropriate foreign elements reveals itself in a strong tendency to assimilate the new to the old, to simplify the manifold, to overlook or repudiate the absolutely contradictory … Its object thereby is the incorporation of new 'experiences' … growth; or more properly, the feeling of growth, the feeling of increased power – is its object. (BGE: 98)

Far from being a structure of inclusion, it is a structure of repudiation, of exclusion, of colonising and dominating the other as the foreign. These features of splitting and exclusion express the assumed separation of diametric space as a movement, combined with the move towards a mirror image inversion of diametric space, in the construction of a power hierarchy of the dominant and the dominated.

Diametric space as mirror image symmetry: the retention of diametric space in Nietzsche's challenge to diametric conceptions of good and evil

A further even more pervasive diametric spatial preoccupation of Nietzsche is with mirror image symmetrical inversion. He offers a litany of inversions that he elevates to a methodology, a conceptual habit of sorts, while noting that he is 'handy at inverting perspectives' (EH: 8), in his oppositional role not as man but as 'dynamite' (EH: 88). These diametric mirror image reversals operate across a range of contrasts he fundamentally relies on, the working–idle caste, higher–lower caste (HH: 211), aristocratic–plebeian, higher dominant race–underrace (GM: 11), clean–unclean (GM: 15), doubt–certainty (EH: 26), heights–abysses (EH: 39), bless–curse (Z: 185), despisers–reverers (Z: 297). Similarly, diametric space as a fragmentation of self into god–demon is observed: '[I]n each ascetic morality, man prays to one part of himself as a god and finds it necessary to diabolify the rest' (HH: 95); these terms import a projected state of mirror image reversal. With cold caverns supporting the glare of the diametric, hierarchies are carved to launch pre-set roles for assimilation.

Stating that: 'Life is a fountain of delight; but where the rabble also drinks all wells are poisoned' (Z: 120), Nietzsche imports a diametric mirror image inversion into life through delight–poison and upper–lower rabble; this is part of the turning against life and its shift towards will to power as hierarchy. In some passages, such as '"Friends, there are no friends!" the dying wise man shouted. "Enemies, there is no enemy! Shout I, the living fool' (HH: 194), Nietzsche develops diametric spatial structures as multiple interlocking mirror image inversions. Elsewhere, he explicitly invokes diametric relations, although not in spatial terms as such, when juxtaposing Greek and Christian deities: 'Grecian gods, these mirrors of noble and grandiose men, in which the animal in man felt itself deified … is diametrically opposed to Christianity's theory of its god' (GM: 64). He explicitly invokes diametric oppositional relations but not as a *spatial* mediating realm impacting on human experience, as well as thought.

Nietzsche's whole reconstruction of morality is imbued with diametric spatial assumptions as mirror image reversals. For example, his deconstruction of the 'good', states that: 'No one has, up to the present, exhibited the faintest doubt or hesitation in judging the "good man" to be of a higher value that the "evil man" … Suppose the converse were the truth! What? Suppose there lurked in the "good man" a symptom of retrogression' (GM: 6). The moralistic constructs of good and bad are treated by Nietzsche as being derivative from a prior set of social relationships between a master and slave class, where a slave morality is 'full of revenge and hate' turned into 'righteousness' (GM: 28).

Again, he seeks to challenge a supposed slave morality, where a view that the wretched are alone good is that of the 'revolt of the slaves' (GM: 17) in morals. This occludes a supposedly noble morality. Again the foundations of morality are for Nietzsche underpinned through a reversal process: '"Who is really evil according to the meaning of the morality of resentment?" … just the good man of the other morality, just the aristocrat, the powerful one, the one who rules, but who is distorted by the venomous eye of resentfulness' (GM: 22). This reversal, as with many of his diametric oppositional hierarchies, is fundamentally linked with will to power, as part of the frontispiece of his argument that morality is a mere plaything of historically constructed power relations –

again a powerful–powerless diametric spatial mirror image reversal operates as a core driving process of his later thought.

An Ariadne thread through his reconstruction of morality is that of diametric space as mirror image inverted symmetry. He conceptualises in terms of compensatory processes that are basically diametric mirror image reversals: '[T]he cardinal moral idea of "ought" originates from the very material idea of "owe" … its origin, in the contractual relationship between *creditor* and *ower*' (GM: 39), so that morality is governed primarily by a commercial principle of reciprocity: 'Sale and purchase, together with their psychological concomitants, are older than the origins of any form of social organisation and union' (GM: 45). This expresses a reciprocal complementarity of figure–ground relation, itself a variant of diametric space as a basic assumed separation. For Nietzsche, the inverted roles between buyer–seller, creditor–owner were part of a quasi-symmetrical process, where the 'individual matched himself against individual' (GM: 45). This is a symmetry as matched reversal of roles, of diametric mirror image symmetry as an exchange process.

Across his work, Nietzsche batters away at the diametric spatial edifice framing the good–bad opposition that he seeks to dismantle stone by stone: 'Good and bad are for a time equivalent to noble and base, master and slave' (HH: 47). *Yet here the more he seeks to break away from the diametric spaces underpinning this, the more he is locked within them in different forms.* Nietzsche diverts and displaces one set of diametric oppositions – good–evil – into another network of diametric spatial relations – master–slave morality, noble–base. The dominion of diametric spatial inverted symmetrical relations is actively sustained even as the content to fill the diametric spatial shells is switched. If he were an actor, Nietzsche would be typecasting himself here in his various roles.

Heidegger highlights the inverted Platonism of Nietzsche's priority for the sensuous realm,[2] as well as the reversal of understanding of art from Schopenhauerian sedative to Nietzschean *stimulans* of life. Heidegger continues: 'But what does that mean – the sensuous stands above all? But as long as the "above and below" define the formal structure of Platonism, Platonism in its essence perdures, the vacant niches of the "above and below" are preserved, suffering only a change in occupancy' (Vol I: 201). However, the above and below are not vacant in another sense, as a relation of diametric space. It is the diametric space that needs overcoming to offer a direct challenge to Platonic metaphysics. Heidegger comments: 'Such overcoming succeeds only when the "above" in general is set aside as such', the apparent world can only be as part of the true'. 'If the true world collapses, so must the world of appearances, But then where does such thinking wind up?' (Vol. I: 201).

Rather than treating Nietzsche's 'perpetual reversal' in pejorative terms as a 'conscious mania', as Heidegger does (Vol. I: 29), Nietzsche's diametric spatial projection of mirror image reversal reveals a profound primordial truth of experience, about the power, scope and primordiality of diametric space as a movement governing experience and life processes.

Diametric space as relative closure

A further feature of diametric space is brought to the fore for Nietzsche's fundamental will of the spirit, namely, closure and noninteraction with background. This further entailment of diametric space is aptly and succinctly described by Nietzsche as follows:

> This same will has at its service an apparently opposed impulse of the spirit, a suddenly adopted preference of ignorance, of arbitrary shutting out, a closing of windows, an inner denial of this or that, a prohibition to approach, a sort of defensive attitude ... the shutting-in horizon. (BGE: 98)

The relative closure of diametric space is epitomised by a 'shutting-in horizon'. The perpetuation of diametric space in later Nietzsche's will to power encompasses a mode of closure to pain (to 'original pain'), combined with a set of mirror image reversals from passive to active, powerless to powerful, love of life (if not other people) to hate and destruction.

Berlin's description of German pietism in the seventeenth and early eighteenth centuries offers an apt description of a wider phenomenon of existential closure as diametric space:

> You gradually hedge yourself round with a kind of tight wall by which you seek to reduce your vulnerable surface – you want to be as little wounded as possible. Every kind of wound has been heaped upon you, and therefore you wish to contract yourself into the smallest possible area, so that as little of you as possible is exposed to further wounds. (2000: 37)

A tightened boundary of exclusion operates both within the diametric spatial structure and in its external relation to environment and is at least briefly apprehended by Nietzsche, although again not in specific spatial structural terms beyond a spatial imagery as a closing of windows and an enclosed horizon.

Diametric space is a tool to that it renders as a tool. The cold skeletal hands of diametric space carve a structure of hard clay that is as much a stamping of lifelessness as a flattening of life into a restricted chamber caging experience – and thereby creating an arbitrary exaltation and relegation within this restricted space.

The dungeon of diametric space operates as a sealed compartment, held together through closure in its very self-definition in opposition to concentric spatial expansion. The dust and soot of diametric space are engrained into walls against permeability, where the clay cold bonds of diametric space cling across experience. Locked doors of diametric space and the stale air of its rooms invade and pervade much of lived experience as will to power.

The mirror image inversion of diametric space as a spatial process of turning: a reversal of life towards destruction

At times, Nietzsche tends to equate the will to power with the will to life, rather than subordinating life to power: '[T]he will itself, the will to power, the unexhausted procreating life-will' (Z: 137), so that the will to power is treated as the zenith of the life principle, with the will to power as 'the strongest and most life-assertive impulse' (GM: 98). Nietzsche treats life as a manifestation not only of power as strength but as an active force of destruction: '[L]ife is essentially (that is in its cardinal functions) something which functions by injuring, oppressing, exploiting and annihilating, and is absolutely inconceivable without such a character' (GM: 49). Yet beyond treating the will to power as a dimension of strength within a life principle, Nietzsche elsewhere treats the will to power as explicitly replacing and subordinating the will to life: '[T]he living creature values many things higher than life itself ... the will to power!' (Z: 138); 'not will to life, but so I teach you – will to power' (Z: 138).

Life is subordinated by Nietzsche not only to a wider principle where 'life is merely a special case of the will to power' (WP: 369), it becomes merely an instrument for this wider principle: 'Life is only a means to something; it is the expression of forms of the growth of power' (WP: 375). In doing so, life turns towards death and cruelty: 'Life itself, its eternal fruitfulness and recurrence, creates torment, destruction, the will to annihilation' (WP: 543), including invocation of 'Dionysus: sensuality and cruelty' (WP: 539) for this assault on a life-giving principle for life.

This replacement and subordination process is a turning process, a turning within life itself: '[L]ife sacrifices itself – for the sake of power!' (Z: 138). Nietzsche here implicitly invokes Dionysus as part of the reconstruction, as power subordinates life, albeit as an internal will or movement within life. As part of this turning process of reversal, 'its life and living beauty grow again out of contempt!' (Z: 154). A diametric mirror image spatial movement of inversion turns life into death, love and beauty into hate and contempt. This is not an accident but a product of a diametric spatial movement, a diametric spatial process of reversal. *The life principle is affected by and embedded interactively in this diametric spatial turning process.*

Nietzsche's will to power is not a mere replacing of the will to life but rather a turning of it, a shift in direction that modifies it, rather than vaporising the will to life. Yet this turn is a radical shift. This is not simply or predominantly a matter of Nietzsche's personal predilection for diametric space as opposition, as mirror image inversion; it is indicative of a wider structural phenomenon, a diametric force as a movement running through life, both as expression of life and as a resistance to it that threatens to submerge life in a further contrary process of destruction of life.

Shelley asks: 'What agencies distinct from life, have acted or act upon life?' (1832/2002: 508). Here, Shelley opens the question that life is itself not a complete system but is impinged on by other forces. Nietzsche can be said to have expanded this insight of Shelley and stretched it to the limit with the counterforce of will to power as diametric space, namely, a spatial system sharing a common domain of interaction with a life drive or spatial movement and yet clashing with life, as an agency distinct from life, while being embedded in life's systemic panorama of movements.

The dominion of diametric space invades Nietzsche's later thought to its core. Against the heat of the passion of Nietzsche's words and the bombastic style, there lurks a cold structure, a moving breathless skeleton of diametric space that marches across the voluminous pages of his thought in a quiet but chilling motion. This is further illustrated through his following observation:

> Perhaps there is no more pregnant principle for any kind of history than the following ... The origin of the existence of a thing and its final utility, its practical application and incorporation into a system of ends, are *toto coelo* opposed to each other – everything, anything, which exists and which prevails anywhere, will always be put to new purposes by a force superior to itself, will be commandeered afresh, will be turned and transformed to new uses; all happening in the organic world consists of *overpowering* and dominating, and again all overpowering and domination is a new interpretation and adjustment, which must necessarily obscure or absolutely extinguish the subsisting meaning and end. (GM: 50)

This is a highly apt description of a Nietzsche's diametric spatial process projected onto life. This diametric mirror image process of reversal, applies directly to his life principle in its turn to will to power, as the end and means for life become inverted and hence subverted.

Observing that 'all ends and utilities are only *signs* that a Will to Power has mastered a less powerful force' (GM: 51), for Nietzsche, life is one of these less powerful forces. With Zarathustra stating that he loves only life most of all when he hates life, again the diametric spatial splitting process serves to split life itself, split its life-giving origins that become subservient to diametrically opposed purposes as the turning to will to power. While recognising Parkes' point that 'Hölderlin's idea of Dionysian *life* that is eternally self-renewing ... deeply impressed Nietzsche just when he was beginning to formulate his first philosophical ideas' (1994: 35), the shift from origin to use brings a diametric opposition to life through power in much of Nietzsche's later work.

Nietzsche explicitly gives the example of punishment as something where 'one identical procedure can be employed and adapted for the most diametrically opposed objects' (GM: 53). He invokes an inversion between origin and utility adopting the explicit language of diametric opposition.[3] Likewise, Nietzsche treats Christianity as having been subjected to a diametric reversal process between origin and function: 'Christianity came into existence in order to lighten the heart; but now it has to burden the heart first' (HH: 87). Where origin is reversed through function, the further step is to envisage this as a specific *spatial* process, a diametric spatial process of inversion.

Nietzsche's account of will to power as experience of a life principle is the actual embodiment of his insight of how origins and functions become diametrically opposed and how functions grow to thwart origins. In other words, Nietzsche's original will to life principle via Schopenhauer, in its origin, has been diametrically inverted, twisted, turned on its head, so that a will to life has become a will to death as a will to power that finds infliction of pain and suffering 'magical', a cardinal function, an end of itself. Whereas suffering facilitates a will to life in Schopenhauer and the Nietzsche of BT, suffering was a means to the end of life; in contrast, in GM, an actual infliction of suffering is elevated into being an end of itself. And, in so doing, life has become the means not its end, power is the end and life, although still extant, has become subordinated. Life has become subordinated as a means to power, as a means to the driving force of diametric space as opposition to life, spreading its dominion over a common domain with life, in a mutually interactive system of relations.

The chain of substitutions in the Nietzschean network is from life to knowledge to power, with the human a means to the superman. This is a diametric mirror image inversion of the will to life. Unlike Foucault's dialectical interplay between power and knowledge where one feeds off the other,[4] the Nietzschean will to power dominates a will to truth: 'Why is knowledge … linked to pleasure ? First and foremost, because by it we gain awareness of our power … any new knowledge … makes us feel superior to *everyone*' (HH: 154). Nietzsche expands on this theme: '*The real philosophers, however, are commanders and law-givers* … Their knowing is creating, their creating is a law-giving, the will to truth is – *Will to Power*' (BGE: 83). They create or construct truths as realities; the will to truth becomes beholden to the will to power, for Nietzsche, again in a monism where one is reduced ultimately to the other in the subordination of truth and knowledge to power.

Where life torments itself to increase knowledge, it appears that knowledge and a will to truth are a superior power to a life principle. Yet elsewhere, it is knowledge that serves a life principle, with the 'importance of knowledge for life' (HH: 17). Diametric mirror image projections again operate between life and knowledge; knowledge is the means to the end of life, although this shifts into a reversal in time becoming life in the service of knowledge.

When asking how much an opinion is 'life-furthering, life-preserving' (BGE: 3) rather than objecting to its falseness, life dominates over truth. Here will to truth is subservient to a life principle, with 'untruth as a condition of life' (BGE: 3). Yet elsewhere Nietzsche goes further with the predominance of knowledge over life as jointly subordinated to the will to power 'your own life takes on the value of a tool and means to knowledge' (HH:175). This occurs as part of reification and instrumentalisation of humanity when treated as an inanimate bridge or rope towards selfovercoming;[5] life becomes a means as a tool, and is here subordinated to knowledge, which is itself characterised as a tool of power. Life becomes a bridge not a goal of itself, a bridge to power.

Again and again, Nietzsche recognises the need to go beyond diametric spatial relations, good–evil. However, repeatedly he displaces his concerns from breaking one kind of diametric relation only to enter into another one. His thought is chained to the diametric space he frequently despises. In Berlin's words, for Schlegel: '[T]he only weapon there is against death … against ossification and against any form of the stabilisation and freezing of the life stream is what he calls *Ironie* … blow it up, point out that the opposite is equally true' (2000: 117). Not only is Nietzsche in the romantic tradition of Schlegel here regarding his use of inversion as a diametric mirror image projection, this process is an injection of movement on a stasis in thought that is to be directly associated with a life movement. This diametric spatial projection as mirror image reversal gives some movement, albeit a limited one.

Nietzsche's pervasive reworking of concepts into a structure of mirror image reversals, his abiding concern to think 'against' and to 'annihilate' are not merely habits of thought or accidental by-products of a fevered imagination or incisive critical acumen. These mirror image inversions offer a distinct projection, a concrete diametric spatial projection, as a dimension of a fundamental orientation in experience projected into thought and language. Yet this fundamental feature of his thought is not explained by him in terms of being a distinct process of experience; Nietzsche is caught in a diametric spatial swamp and it is the air he breathes but frequently does not appear to know how to modify or emerge from. This projection is of a fundamental primordial experience, a living manifestation and embodiment of the very will to power that Nietzsche acutely describes as a basic conceptual foundation of his later work. Yet this conceptual habit of thought is underpinned by a distinct experiential projection of diametric space.[6]

A later Nietzschean vista is one where the life principle becomes a mere vassal to the will to power; a will to life principle is turned into sheer raw material for the enthronement of the will to power. These accounts are not simply a Nietzschean frenzy; they give expression to a concrete spatial systemic process underpinning experience, a fundamental dynamic of diametric spatial movements colonising experiential space. Much of the diametric spatial rush to inversion in Nietzsche's account of the will to power, underpinned by the switch away from diametric constructs of good and evil, can be interpreted as an *alienation* of the will to life through the will to power. This is not an alienation as falsity but rather a subversion, loss, pollution or degradation of the concentric will to life force, as it is subjected to a turning process of diametric space. Alienation here in spatial terms refers to a process prior to the Marxist notion of reification that operates within a subject–object dualism (and understanding of alienated labour in capitalism). Alienation here means a twisting from concentric space to diametric space, to a reified diametric space as a conditioning environment of distance to give rise to the subject–object mode, as a precondition for objectness; the *Gegenstand* of objectness is a diametric spatial standing opposite, standing against. This alienation as reification connotes a loss of life in the fall from concentric to diametric relations, even if this foreground diametric structure may be a helpful reaction in some systemic circumstances.

The life flow enters a space of reification that opposes and divides it – a diametric space. This turns life against itself, through a subversion and alienation process that is one of mirror image inversion. On this view of diametric space as alienation, diametric space is an interactive expression of injury to concentric space, as a by-product of concentric space. Diametric space is also a violence on concentric space, as a process of infliction, a power that fractures the flow of concentric structured spatial relations.

Will to power in the *Nachlass* places *interpretation* centrally. Such a perspectivism, as the relativity of perspectives in a power hierarchy, is built into the structure of diametric space, with its mirror image inversions to include the powerful and powerless. Yet diametric spaces move at a different level, prior to cognition as interpretation; this will to power as diametric space is at a different level from interpretation but nevertheless, affects the *framing conditions* for interpretation.

A perspectivism, as the relativity of perspectives in a power hierarchy, is built into the structure of diametric space. The operation of diametric space is primarily prior to the *cogito*, it moves at a different level, yet in doing so it affects the framing conditions for interpretation. In this sense, the will to power is interpretative as Nietzsche notes, regarding its power to create:

> [T]he will to power interprets (it is a question of interpretation when an organ is constructed): it defines limits, determines degrees, variations of power … there must be present something that wants to grow and interprets the value of whatever else wants to grow … interpretation is itself a means of becoming master of something (the organic process constantly presupposes interpretations). (WP: 342)

It is a movement that engages with the environment, establishing relations in the environment, including boundaries and this engagement is an interpretation as such.

Ames' words are apposite here, to recognise that this is not a sheer relativity of any kind of perspectivism: 'Nietzsche posits the notion of "power" to provide a standard that distinguishes his aesthetic perspectivism from anything goes relativism. Will to power is the drive to interpret and hence "create" a world on one's own terms' (1991: 145). However, Ames' position here appears to be an anthropocentric view of will to power. This is apt for a foreground will to power in lived experience but not for the background diametric space as will to power, which is a wider cosmological principle, pertaining also to impact on a life principle and affecting structural conditions for lived experience.

Will to power is not simply subjectivist but pertaining to a life domain beyond the human subject. It is to be emphasised that the will to power as an extension of Schopenhauer's will to life is an unconscious transsubjective driving force, even if Nietzsche subsequently rejects a metaphysical will in itself, Schopenhauer's will is 'a mere empty word' (WP: 369). Nietzsche also rejects will as sheer subjectivism: '[T]he will of psychology … *does not exist at all*' (WP: 369).

Without needing to share a conception of virtue as a static trait, Copleston's observation that it is 'a great mistake to suppose that mere power is the sole Nietzschean virtue' (1942/1975: 83) offers an important insight. He continues: '[I]f power were really the one value in Nietzsche's eyes, it should follow that the victorious and reigning herd is justified … But Nietzsche constantly and fiercely inveighs against herd-morality, herd-valuation, herd-supremacy, he will not allow that the mediocre majority are entitled to restrain the strong and freespirited individuals' (1942/1975: 82). As a cosmological principle of will as a variant of will to life, will to power requires a systemic description prior to simple human subjectivity. Yet it is also expressed as a systemic force in the experience of the individual; both levels of description require reconciliation, as well as distinction from the level of description of the group as herd. Will to power is being interpreted here as both a spatial-phenomenological principle affecting the individual's experience and as a wider cosmological system principle, in the world beyond simple human subjectivity.

While will to power may be expressed through subjective wills, it is primarily an impersonal movement, a system propagating itself. The will to power as a dynamic system of diametric spatial relations feeding off themselves moves this away from being beholden to sheer subjectivism or vulnerable to the accusations of Heidegger that this is still a naive ground for the subject that is part of a Western metaphysics of substituting one ground/centre for another. This diametric spatial movement as will to power is not an atomic structuralist foundation, such as a Cartesian *cogito* but is rather a systemic propagation and movement.[7]

Heidegger treats Nietzsche as the last metaphysician, trapped within a metaphysics of subjectivity in the will to power and in a substitute of one fundamental ground for another as a kind of fundamental substance. Yet will to power as diametric space is neither tethered to subjectivity as a transpersonal systemic process and movement, nor is it a substance as such; it is a relation, a relational medium of space that is not an entity as an object. It is a precondition for objecthood and substance.

This is not to deny that at times Nietzsche constructs the will in terms open to the accusation of simple subjectivity, for example, where referring to 'a will for Nothingness, a will opposed to life, but it is and remains *a will*! …

man will wish *Nothingness* rather than not wish *at all*' (GM: 118). This emphasis on will as active control, subsequently amplified by Freud (1920), is will as mere subjectivity and a subdimension of wider diametric spatial mirror image inversion of active/passive will; it is here vulnerable to Heidegger's critique of subjective will as metaphysics. Nevertheless, individual consciousness of power is but one aspect under the umbrella of the diametric space of the will to power.

A feature of the power principle, for Nietzsche, is how inextricably related it is to the life principle; one appears together with the other, as a turn within the other, although typically a unidirectional turn from life to power, with little on a reciprocal turning process from power to life. *It is this turn to life from diametric spatial power that opens up a potential space for concentric spatial movement as a structural modification of the diametric.*

Diametric space in the historical myth of Dionysus

With Nietzsche as the self-proclaimed 'disciple of the philosopher Dionysus' (EH: 3), the Dionysian myth requires further exploration to apprehend the full reach of its betrothal to diametric space. The will to power can be treated as a firmer expression of Dionysian principles once the full force of the historical accounts of Dionysian sacrifices, somewhat underplayed by Nietzsche in BT, are recognised, as evinced in Kerenyi's historical overview for the Dionysian in ancient Greece. Whereas Heidegger's neglect of the Dionysian features of Nietzsche's thought is well known (Krell 1991), Heidegger combines this neglect with his prioritisation of Nietzsche's so-called doctrine of eternal recurrence over will to power. Recognition of the importance of the Dionysian for understanding Nietzsche's thought, especially with regard to will to power, is not intended to foreground will to power over eternal recurrence. Neither is it to overlook changing emphases between Nietzsche's account of the Dionysian in his early and later works. The question of the relation between will to power and eternal recurrence will be considered subsequently in Chapter 8.

In Kerenyi's detailed and authoritative historical account of the Dionysian myth in ancient Greece, diametric mirror image inversions and splitting dominate, to an even greater degree than in Nietzsche's account in BT. These are evident in the details of the Dionysian festivals' activities and sacrifices, the compensatory function of atonement displayed in these rituals, as well as the structure of the temporal changes; the two-year phase of the Dionysian year imports a diametric spatial inversion of absence and presence, times when the Dionysian is expected to arrive and times when it is absent. Initial examples of diametric mirror image inversion include the dancers around the enthroned in the Dionysian festival are treated as both murderers and saviours, with the sacrifice being of god's representative *and* enemy:

> If the dancers had not previously danced around the child Dionysus in order, seemingly, to kill him, it would be impossible to understand how they could cease to be the child's saviors, as they were elsewhere in Greek mythology, and become his murderers. The development is from less humane to more humane gods, not the reverse. Ceasing to be murderers, they became saviors. (Kerenyi 1976: 266)

With echoes of the fraternal bond between Dionysus and Apollo, proposed by Nietzsche in BT, Kerenyi quotes Otto on what amounts to a mirror image bond as a sibling relationship *within* the Dionysian:

> The vine and the ivy are like siblings who have developed in opposite directions and yet cannot deny their relationship. Both undergo an amazing metamorphosis. In the cool season of the year the vine lies as though dead and in its dryness resembles a useless stump until the moment when it feels the renewed heat of the sun and blossoms forth in a riot of green … What happens in the ivy is no less remarkable. Its cycle of growth gives evidence of a duality which is quite capable of suggesting the two-fold nature of Dionysus.[8] (1965: 153–155)

A further diametric spatial feature of the Dionysian rites is that of splitting. The diametric splitting involves the destruction and tearing asunder of the sacrificial animal. The bull is torn to pieces as a characterisation of the suffering dismembered god of Dionysus. On Kerenyi's accounts, the Dionysian ritual sacrifice involves a cutting out of the heart or phallus from the sacrificial animal, as part of the phallic procession. Kerenyi is clear on the cruelty ('cruel sacrifice') of these rituals, which also included at times tearing a sacrificial child to pieces, 'the infant Dionysus, like the sacrificed kid, was first boiled and then roasted' (1976: 247); 'These occasions, their feast days, must be regarded as realizations of aggressive, murderous life' (1976: 85). The cruelty in the historical Dionysian rituals in ancient Greece is directly confronted by Kerenyi: '[T]he sacrificial animal was dismembered, something was set aside and kept' (1976: 259); 'It was not a heart but a phallus' (1976: 260). This was 'a cruel death, a repetition of the rending of Dionysus; such a death was re-enacted, probably in a very much abbreviated and simplified form, in each sacrifice of a goat' (Kerenyi 1976: 235). Kerenyi continues:

> The bull games of the Cretans were a continuation of the bull capture, enacted in the form of a drama. It seems hardly credible that in a wild Dionysus cult such powerful animals should have been torn to pieces alive by the teeth of the participants and devoured raw, but we have express testimony showing that this monstrous rite occurred in a feast of Dionysus repeated every two years. (1976: 84)

The function of this diametric splitting process was again a diametric one of mirror image inversion as a compensation, a compensatory atonement through the sacrifice for the killing of Dionysus as a child; 'the somber Dionysian sacrifice, the murder of the god' (Kerenyi 1976: 243) is compensated for in mirror image reverse symmetry fashion through the sacrificial animal, 'a substitutive sacrifice presupposing the identity of god, man and animal – a sacrifice characteristic of the Dionysian religion' (1976: 236). Likewise, Ivanov observes the Dionysian as importing the identification of the god with both the sacrifice and the sacrificed, which is again a diametric spatial relation as mirror image reversal. Kerenyi continues: 'Two objects pertaining to the historical Dionysus cult, the mask and the goat, appear on a stone seal in a tomb near Phaistos: the mask is manifestation of the god, and the goat (a characteristic sacrificial animal of the Dionysian religion) is his substitute' (1976: 80).

As a compensatory atonement, the goat is in a diametric mirror image relation to the god and mask as god manifestation. In contrast, concentric space offers no such recompense; it is not within the borders of a compensatory reversal such as that of the diametric space of inversion. The function of atonement, of a kind of debtor–creditor relationship, is one of a diametric mirror image inversion. Otherness as substitute is within the diametric structure of sacrifice for atonement. This is scarcely a structure of inclusion of the other.

Ivanov remarks on the 'many contrary principles that are reconciled in Dionysian religion, solemn weeping and unbridled laughter, sacrifice and dance, the ivy of winter and the rose of spring' (quoted and translated in West 1970: 78). Much depends on the conception of reconciliation. A diametric spatial mirror image symmetry holds contrary principles together in a common structured relation, yet this is far from an active reconciliation, but is more a dynamic tension. Such oppositional tension gives expression to a figure–ground relation as a variant of diametric space. However, these relations do not offer a structural reconciliation but rather hold both domains separately in a diametric space of assumed separation without mutual transformation; there is no restructuring of mutual boundaries to bring an assumed connection of concentric space.

Dionysus as a life-bearing principle is, in Kerenyi's words, turned to death through the sacrificial rites. Again this is a diametric mirror image reversal. Moreover, Kerenyi refers to the 'subterranean Dionysus' (1976: 289) as a reversal of life itself. The dual aspect of Dionysus, recognised explicitly by Kerenyi, is that of protector of life and killer of life in death. Kerenyi described this ritual realisation in Dionysian festivals: 'The murder of the Divine Child was his reduction to an organ from which – or as which – he could be reawakened' (1976: 267). This led to 'phallus processions and merry Dionysian festivals … held throughout the Greek countryside' for the Dionysus of the Athenians (1976: 285), 'the protector of life', 'the lord of all living creatures' (1976: 323). These ritual sacrifices betray a clear diametric mirror image inversion structure – including a shift from passive receipt of the death of the child

Dionysus to active perpetration of death of a sacrificial animal or child in the Dionysian rites. The community exerts a power over the suffering, even through its diametric structured mirror image ambivalence of concern and aggression towards the sacrificial animal, whether he-goat, bull or indeed child.

The will to power, as with the dual-sidedness of the Dionysian cults and myths, accommodates a life principle within a wider principle of power to negate this principle, in an overall diametric spatial projection of inverted symmetry. The diametric spatial projection of inversion through Dionysian atonement is the shift from passive suffering to active infliction of suffering and killing as part of the will to power. The will to power subsumes the will to life as an element within its wider systemic propagation.

While Kerenyi also supports the view of Dionysian as 'overflowing life' (1976: 252), the sacrificial kill as the turning of the will to life plays itself out in the Dionysian narrative built on diametric spatial relations. In Kerenyi's words:

> The god who goads them on is the opposite of what he was in the first year, the opposite of him who roused beings to life, of the lord of the dead who wants to be awakened. Now he is the lord of all living creatures who drives them to kill and in the death of the slain is so reduced that he is in need of awakening. Dionysus is the quarry of the hunt and the sacrificial animal, both of which are eaten raw. (1976: 203)

Embedded once again in a diametric system of meaning as mirror image reversals, life turns to death, as does the life principle under the hegemony of the will to power.

Freud's (1920) account of ritual as not only revealing of obsessional neurosis but also a compulsion to repeat, giving expression to a death drive, gains support from these accounts. Significantly, for current purposes, Freud (1920) emphasises another feature of such rituals resonant with a diametric spatial projection, namely, the *closed* ritual of the sacrifice as a compulsion to repeat; this closure into a defensive shell bears further hallmarks of diametric space. It is additional to the diametric mirror image feature of the rituals' compensatory function, as a compensatory mirror image atonement in the shift from passivity towards being an active protagonist. The diametric spatial features of opposition, active splitting and mirror image compensatory atonement and power hierarchies all support Freud's characterisation of the death drive.[9] Kerenyi quotes Otto: 'No single Greek god even approaches Dionysus in the horror of his epithets, which bear witness to a savagery that is absolutely without mercy … surely there can be no further doubt that this puts us into death's sphere' (1965: 113). This raises the question at least of diametric space underpinning major features of the Dionysian rituals as giving expression to a death drive, at least in the sense of Freud's active process of destruction.

Kerenyi explicates a dual reversal dimension of ambivalence: '[T]he two statues stood for festivals of two kinds: one centering on the apparent slaying and mutilation of the god and the real slaying of his representative, the kid; the other expressing joy at the happy end of the somber action that had been performed a year before' (1976: 323); 'the sacrifice … a highly ambivalent action of which people did not like to speak' (1976: 251). Ambivalence is the epitome of a diametric spatial–relational mirror image splitting projection.

Parkes highlights the mask-related feature of the game of the Dionysian duality: 'The duplex being of Dionysus governs the various dualities of the mask as bidirectional mediator between self and other, inside and outside' (1994: 340), including self-deception and of others. This is again amenable to interpretation in terms of diametric space as mirror image reversal. Moreover, as Kerenyi explicates: 'When the trieteris was replaced by the one year period – a process probably completed in the sixth century – the sad and joyful elements were combined in a complex game' (1976: 323). Nietzsche's twist is that there is also a sadistic happiness in the cruelty, a revelling in the cruelty as an end in itself. Kerenyi highlights the systemic 'logic' to the Dionysian ritual: 'The Dionysian sacrificial rite with its complex structure and strict inner logic was one of the basic facts of Greek religious history' (1976: 261). The further step here is to characterise this 'game' as a diametric spatial systemic logic.

Nietzsche's will to life through Dionysian (prelinguistic) music may retain its features of excess, sexual transgression, intoxication but these have turned against their prior cardinal function to serve life as will to life, to be an 'optic of life' (BT: 5). Now they are an optic of power in all its diametric spatial forms – these diametric spatial modes are a turning towards death. A killing of the life pulse, a pulsating life that Nietzsche saw in a fusion of pleasure and pain that again retains a notion of pleasure and with it pain; while pleasure and pain as ends of themselves remain intact, nevertheless, pleasure and pain now serve a different function from will to life in their turn against this into will to power.

The Dionysian rituals give lucid expression to Freud's death drive as a diametric spatial propagation, involving a compulsion to repeat, ritual compensatory defences as obsessional neuroses to avenge the killing of the Dionysian child – as mirror image reversals – as destruction in a closed ritual space of repetition, involving a range of diametric mirror image relations.[10] It is difficult to disavow a reading of such Dionysian sacrificial rites in terms not only of Freud's treatment of religious rituals as obsessional neuroses, but also as expression of the compulsion to repeat and the aggressive drive to destroy both of which Freud integrated into a conception of Thanathos, the death drive, an optic of death. These Dionysian sacrifices are defence mechanisms against *passively* experiencing death through an *active* killing, a diametric mirror image reversal between being active and passive that is again a feature of Freud's compulsion to repeat as a hallmark of the death drive (see Downes 2012).

Nietzsche's turning within the will to life is thoroughly consistent with his earlier positions as an extension of the primacy of the Dionysian principle. While Nietzsche may be criticised for his *celebration* of a diametric space as a will to power, the accuracy of his description is not to be contested. He can be criticised for failing to bring to further light the diametric spatial processes underpinning this shift in the life principle. He observes the twisting and inversion of an origin principle from a purpose, but he does not explain this in terms of diametric *spatial* movements. Nietzsche is blinded to the spatial features and this spatial medium for the processes he describes, through his prior epistemological commitment to treating space as merely an ephemeral construct of mind without being a more fundamental reality at the level of the will in itself as a directional movement. In other words, it is Nietzsche's Kantian and Schopenhauerean commitments *regarding space* that occlude his perception of the fundamentally spatial features of the diametric processes he acutely observes.

Against this historical backdrop for the Dionysian myth, it is evident that the blithe equation of a Dionysian life principle with Schopenhauer's will to life in BT must be called into question, as Kerenyi also does.[11] It would be more apt to interpret the Dionysian myth as expounded by Kerenyi in terms of the will to power of Nietzsche rather than flatly as a will to life principle.

Nietzsche's mirror image diametric spatial projections are far from being an accidental by-product of this thought, they are not only selfconsciously included as a proud methodological invertor of opposites but also they are deeply imbued in his self-proclaimed role as a disciple of Dionysus. In other words, the Dionysian myth is replete with this diametric spatial structure of mirror image inversions, closure and splits. Thus, Nietzsche can be said to be embodying the Dionysian not only in the content of this thought but in its very structure – a structure of splitting and ambivalence, as a diametric mirror image projection on the panoply of dimensions across which he casts his cold eye and being.

Will to power: hemiplegia of the connective will

Nietzsche's amplification of the will to power as a turning within the will to life, in Dionysian terms, is strongly consistent with the Dionysian myth to build in features given less emphasis in BT. However, this consistency still betrays a fundamental flaw in much of Nietzsche's corpus of work, the lack of capacity for conceptual understanding of the opposite directional space to the diametric spatial projections he persistently propagates, namely, concentric directional space. This rigidity in Nietzsche's position amounts to a calcification in his experience and thought as his reasoning processes virtually assume that life is to be equated with the diametric space he projects, so that anything that challenges this becomes, by definition, antithetical to life. Nevertheless, challenge to diametric space does not mean being engaged in an antithesis to life itself.

While Nietzsche repeatedly distances his positions from Darwinism, Nietzsche's life as will to power offers much resonance with a Hobbesian life as a state of war as a vehicle of nature, a life nasty, brutish and short. Nietzsche's timorous retreat from connection, from the embedded web of concentric relation of space is a brute reduction to diametric space; it is a reduction that is not without empirical support as one dimension of reality as life, but to the extent that it occludes a further possibility of concentric space of assumed connection, it is a sheer neglect of empirical actuality as well as of experiential possibility.[12]

Later Nietzschean thought is ravaged by diametric space, all the while that he seeks to ravage the conceptual foundations of Western thought, in search of a reevaluation of values. If Joyce's *Dubliners* were beset by what he termed a 'hemiplegia of the will', Nietzsche's life principle becomes ridden with a *hemiplegia of the connective will.* With Nietzsche's flight from connection, from the assumed connection of concentric space, a loss arises, a loss of the quiver of fragility as a pulse of connective vitality. The shell consumes the egg, the riverbank consumes the river. It is not unfair to conclude that for Nietzsche, hell is not so much other people as *connection with* other people, and its related unfolding of vulnerability to dissolve a will to power. Nietzsche bemoans where 'weakness is turned to merit' (GM: 27), while rejecting an understanding of shared mutual expression of vulnerability as a distinctively human strength, key for human wellbeing. With his reliance on the will to power as the ultimate driving principle and a commitment to appearance that allows for no veils, Nietzsche sees the foreground scab of diametric space, but not the flow as underlying blood of concentric space; he perceives the frozen ice of diametric space, but not the movement of water flow of concentric space.

Dionysian 'joy' amounts to the reinstantiation and replication of diametric space, as a membrane of remembrance. This function of preservation and expansion of the dominion of diametric space in the Dionysian as will to power differs quite dramatically from earlier Nietzsche's rapture as expression of the Dionysian. Early Nietzsche's prerepresentational rapture is a transgression of the already excessive, as an addition to the sheer historical manifestations of the Dionysian myth in ancient Greece. However, arguably Nietzsche's projective gloss on the historical Dionysian with rapture goes further; it can be interpreted as a structural modification of the Dionysian. It offers a restructuring of the very mode of the Dionysian to enter another space of experience. It does not serve the function of preservation and celebration of diametric space but does the opposite; it subverts diametric space, whether in the direction of a monistic fusion with background stimuli or towards the lost scent of a concentric spatial direction for experiential restructuring.

Although Nietzsche asks where is the 'opposed will' 'opponent ideal' to asceticism (GM: 111), he never directly asks where is the opposed counterpole to the diametric spatial projections he perpetually engages in as his default operation and approach to life and reasoning as will to power.[13] The will to power appears as a conceptual monism for Nietzsche. This invites a question as to what is the opposition to opposition itself as will to power. Nietzsche fails to ask this selfreferential question, at least explicitly, although a case can be made (see Chapter 8) that eternal recurrence is an implicit response to this question. Hence he loses or never directly grasps sight of a prior movement or struggle – that is, he does not directly apprehend the power struggle itself between the will to power as diametric space and a contrary pole of concentric space as inclusion, connection and openness. The sole *modus vivendi* of struggle for Nietzsche is one of annihilation, breaking, splitting; thus, he overlooks the power struggle between breaking as a solid splitting and dissolving as a fluid restructuring that encompasses, that includes. This power struggle between diametric breaking and concentric dissolving operates at different levels, as a foreground, background and projection of fragments of this struggle into concrete life contexts and systemic worlds.[14] The question now arises as to whether will to power can also embrace concentric spatial relations as another dimension pertaining to a life principle, and in so doing, address *another power tension*, namely, that *between diametric space and concentric space* in their ongoing interplay.

This wider scope of questioning for the will to power operates not simply within diametric space and its power hierarchy. Is there a diametric spatial relation or concentric spatial relation *between* diametric and concentric spaces? [15]

This wider question is not confined to will to power *within* diametric space but *between* diametric and concentric spaces. It is less than clear that Nietzsche directly addresses this wider will to power question. Arguably it is the wider lens of eternal recurrence, related to will to power but not to be simply equated with will to power that offers the scope for interaction between concentric and diametric spaces and hence a wider questioning in relation to will to power.

Despite Nietzsche's repeated exhortations to dance, 'to dance on the feet of chance' (Z: 186) and what he elsewhere observes as a difference between dancing and staggering[16] – the Nietzschean dance of the will to power is a dance on one foot, solely on the sole of diametric space. In other words, later Nietzsche staggers into the primordial terrain of diametric space, without any apparent avenue for exiting it into a wider expanse of concentric spatial movements. Where can this avenue be found?

Notes

1 Berlin treats power as the central concern of, for example, the late eighteenth-century and early nineteenth-century thinker Maistre, explicitly perceiving a resonance with Nietzsche (2003: 151–153).

2 As Parkes also emphasises, Plato's and Nietzsche's 'projects are in one sense diametrically opposed: the former's being to purify the psyche of all earthly accretions, the latter's to redeem its somatic aspect for the earth' (1994: 184). Moreover, as Parkes

argues, the conclusion of Zarathustra's speech offers an 'erotic inversion of the climax of the discourse Diotima delivers to Socrates' (1994: 236).

3 Berlin characterises this inversion of origin and impact as a feature of romanticism: 'The result of romanticism ... is liberalism, toleration, decency and the appreciation of the imperfections of life ... Aiming at one thing, they produced, fortunately for us all, almost the exact opposite' (2000: 147).

4 For Foucault, 'the exercise of power perpetually creates knowledge and, conversely, knowledge constantly induces effects of power' (1980: 52).

5 'Man is a rope, fastened between animal and Superman – a rope over an abyss' (Z: 43), 'a bridge not a goal' (Z: 44).

6 Concentric and diametric spaces are structures of difference in relation to self and other. This invites a Derridean questioning (Downes 2012, 2013). Derrida (1985) interrogates projections of embodied experience into language and thought, to go beyond the Platonic priority given to the visual. Hence he deconstructs texts for example, to uncover the ear of the other and the haptic. This approach to interrogating fundamental experiential projections into texts is taken a step further here in relation to primordial experiences of spatial relations to self and world that are prior to the five senses, for example, experience of breathing, of the breath (Downes 2012), resonant with a long tradition of associating breath with spirit. It is these concentric and diametric primordial breath spaces for experience that are unwittingly projected into texts, including Nietzsche's seminal concepts. While these breath experiences may be experienced selfconsciously, they need not be selfconsciously experienced to operate as projections, as projected structures of difference.

7 See Dreyfus and Rabinow (1982) on holistic structuralism in contrast to atomistic structuralism, a distinction expanded on in Downes (2012).

8 Otto continues: 'First it puts out the so-called shade-seeking shoots, the scandent tendrils with the well-known lobed leaves. Later, however, a second knot of shoot appears which grows upright and turns toward the light. The leaves are formed completely differently and now the plant produces flowers and berries. Like Dionysus, it could well be called the 'twice-born'. But the way in which it produces its flowers and fruit is both strikingly similar to and yet startlingly different from that found in the vine. It blooms, namely, in the autumn, when the grapes of the vine are harvested. And it produces its fruit in spring. Between its blooming and its fruiting lies the time of Dionysus' epiphany in the winter months ... While the vine of Dionysus needs as much light and heat from the sun as it can get, the ivy of Dionysus has surprisingly little need for light and warmth, and grows green and fresh in the shade and in the cold too' (1965: 153–155).

9 See Downes (2012) for development of this argument in more detail, including concentric space in terms of a life drive of Freud.

10 As Kerenyi observes: 'Throughout Greek and Roman antiquity the custom of sacrificing a goat to the vine remained in force. The sacrifice was explained by a kind of law of *talion*, for when goats were admitted to a vineyard they sinned against the vines. "So it came about", says Marcus Terentius Varro, "that the he-goats were sacrificed to Dionysus, discoverer of the vine, as though to make atonement, a head for a head"' (1976: 249). This is significant for making explicit the compensatory atonement function of the sacrifice, a mirror image relation in the law of *talion*. The cult itself is a closed group in a closed system of diametric spatial closure. Freud's ritual sacrifice as obsessional neurosis, involves a compulsion to repeat 'the killing of Dionysus, which was to be repeated in Perinthos in the form of a sacrifice' (1976: 251). This invokes a diametric spatial mode of a passive–active shift as instantiation of the will to power. Dionysus is sacrificed and then requires sacrificial atonement, as a passive–active interplay of diametric mirror image reversal.

11 This is quite apart from debates resting on the malleability and historical evolution of Dionysian myths where the Dionysian is situated by Nietzsche as antichristian and elsewhere as an embodiment of the Christian myth (Ivanov, in West 1970).
12 The position taken up here, on the will to power specifically, does not share Stambaugh's position where she states: 'I believe that Nietzsche implicitly places the affirmation of life at the center of man's being' (1994: 9).
13 Singh treats Schopenhauer as being trapped in an either–or mode regarding asceticism as a full denial of the will and a 'thoughtless and ongoing affirmation of the will-to-live' (2016: 44) that is tantamount to a cage of diametric space.
14 Concentric space as dissolving is far removed from the advocacy of 'sculpting' of self by Bishop (2017), invoking both Nietzsche and Jung; it is not a selfshaping through the selfconscious ego but rather a self-opening to levels prior to familiar ego consciousness. Will to power is not simply interpretative, although also operating at such a level. As a primordial diametric spatial movement, it is precognitive and not simply anthropocentric.
15 This question enters the terrain of Heidegger's questioning of the horizon of relation between being and nonbeing, and Freud's tensions between life and death drives (see Downes 2012).
16 'Dancing is not the same thing as staggering wearily back and forth between different impulses' (HH: 169).

References

Ames, R. T., 'Nietzsche's "Will to Power" and Chinese "Virtuality" (De): A Comparative Study', in G. Parkes (ed.), *Nietzsche and Asian Thought.* Chicago, IL: University of Chicago Press, 1991.

Berlin, I., *The Roots of Romanticism. The A. W. Mellon Lectures in the Fine Arts, 1965. The National Gallery of Art, Washington, DC.* Henry Hardy (ed.). London: Pimlico, 2000.

Berlin, I., *Freedom and Its Betrayal. Six Enemies of Human Liberty.* H. Hardy (ed.). London: Pimlico, 2003.

Bishop, P., *On the Blissful Islands with Nietzsche and Jung.* London: Routledge, 2017.

Copleston, F., *Friedrich Nietzsche: Philosopher of Culture.* New York: Barnes & Noble Books, 1942/1975.

Derrida, J., *The Ear of the Other: Otobiography, Transference, Translation.* C. V. MacDonald (ed.), trans. P. Kamuf. New York: Schocken Books, 1985.

Downes, P., *The Primordial Dance: Diametric and Concentric Spaces in the Unconscious World.* Oxford/Bern: Peter Lang, 2012.

Downes, P., 'Developing Derrida's Psychoanalytic Graphology: Diametric and Concentric Spatial Movements', *Derrida Today*, 2013, 6(2): 197–221.

Dreyfus, H. L. and Rabinow, P., *Michel Foucault: Beyond Structuralism and Hermeneutics.* New York: Harvester Wheatsheaf, 1982.

Foucault, M., 'Prison Talk', in C. Gordon (ed.), *Power/Knowledge.* Harlow: Prentice Hall, 1980.

Frankopan, P., *The Silk Roads: A New History of the World.* London: Bloomsbury, 2015.

Freud, S., *Beyond the Pleasure Principle.* SE 18. London: Hogarth Press, 1920.

Heidegger, M., *Nietzsche*, Vols I and II. D. F. Krell (ed.), trans. D. F. Krell. New York: HarperCollins, 1991.

Kerenyi, C., *Dionysus: Archetypal Image of Indestructible Life.* Princeton, NJ: Princeton University Press, 1976.

Krell, D. F., 'Introduction to the Paperback Edition', in M. Heidegger, *Nietzsche* Vols I and II. D. F. Krell (ed.), trans. D. F. Krell. New York: HarperCollins, 1991, ix–xxvii.

Otto, W. F., *Dionysus: Myth and Cult*. Trans. R. B. Palmer. London: Bloomington, 1965.

Parkes, G., *Composing the Soul: Reaches of Nietzsche's Psychology*. Chicago, IL: University of Chicago Press, 1994.

Shelley, P. B., 'Mont Blanc', in D. H. Reiman and N. Fraistat (eds.), *Shelley's Poetry and Prose*. New York: W. W. Norton, 1817/2002, 97–101.

Shelley, P. B., 'The Triumph of Life', in D. H. Reiman and N. Fraistat (eds.), *Shelley's Poetry and Prose*. New York: W. W. Norton, 1822/2002, 483–500.

Shelley, P. B., 'On Life', in D. H. Reiman and N. Fraistat (eds.), *Shelley's Poetry and Prose*. New York: W. W. Norton, 1832/2002, 505–509.

Singh, R. R., *Death, Contemplation and Schopenhauer*. New York: Routledge, 2016.

Stambaugh, J., *The Other Nietzsche*. New York: State University of New York Press, 1994.

West, J., *Russian Symbolism: A Study of Vyacheslav Ivanov and the Russian Symbolist Aesthetic*. London: Methuen, 1970.

Chapter 7

Space as freedom in experience

Differing Dionysian visions and conceptions of bounded freedom in Nietzsche's work

In a move beyond diametric space, are there seeds of concentric space to be located? The Dionysian myth in its multifarious manifestations[1] and different emphases glue together the earlier and later Nietzschean corpus and while there is a turn against life in the later from the earlier, this is far from being a turn against the Dionysian. What is of most interest from the perspective of exploration of a life-giving concentric spatial principle, is the appendage onto the Dionysian in early Nietzsche (Kerenyi's 'fairy tale' 1976: 135, for Nietzsche's account) namely, the enchantment of the portrayed unity in experience as part of apprehension of imageless experience in music. The extra layer of coating added on to the Dionysian in early Nietzsche tells more about the existential experiential features of Nietzsche than if this addendum were omitted as part of a sheer textual fidelity to historical factual accounts of the Dionysian.

One reading of Nietzsche's modification of the will to life in its turn towards the primacy of the will to power is that Nietzsche has in some way lost his prior Dionysian insights regarding fluidity as a loosening and opening in experience, implicating concentric space. While Nietzsche's turn towards the will to power as the driving force prior even to the will to life, as a turning of the will to life, is a loss of potential avenues for concentric space in his earlier thought, it is not a loss of the Dionysian; the concentric dimensions of an experiential opening were a projective excess upon the historical Dionysus. In contrast, the will to power is the full-fledged expression of his earlier Dionysian vision. It not only gives expression to his insight that origins turn against functions. It also requires recognition that diametric spatial assumptions thoroughly saturate the Dionysian myth. Will to power as diametric space is far from being 'a paltry subject' as characterised by Bataille (1945: 85); it is a fundamental primordial space, as diametric spatial movements.

The umbrella term of the Dionysian is used by Nietzsche to conflate the rapture of music in BT with the different rapture of the sacrificial ritual, with its killings and dances as will to power. The rapture of music as overcoming the *principium individuationis* is an appendage projected onto the Dionysian myth by early Nietzsche without historical justification and via Schopenhauer's insight. The apparent threads of commonality between these forms of rapture need to be unravelled through dismantling their unity in the Dionysian construct, building on Nietzsche's own disdain for forced unities. This is not an argument for a further duality within the Dionysian as two masks each from the other. It is rather to treat the latter Dionysian in Nietzsche's thought as a diametric spatial system of will to power and the former Dionysian in Nietzsche as inviting a diametrically opposed goal, namely, to reach beyond diametric spatial boundaries of the *principium individuationis*. This earlier reaching beyond diametric space can be interpreted as fusion with background into a monism, with steps also towards a concentric spatial opening. This spatial-phenomenological reading of Nietzsche in terms of diametric and concentric spatial projections takes Nietzsche at least partly beyond the apparel of the Dionysian. The Dionysian is a largely unhelpful façade for Nietzsche's important experiential projections in BT, although the Dionysian is a vital framework for will to power, as a multidimensional diametric spatial system, in his later work.

While Nietzsche does not advocate a conception of freedom as a creativity *ex nihilo*, as some kind of subjective will *causa sui*, multiple multifaceted conceptions of freedom can emerge from interpretation of his work, including, for example, the proposed transformation of the soul in Zarathustra from camel to lion to child or the epicurean vision in the GS. There is also the question of how even a bounded freedom can be sustained if the implications of his later exploration of eternal recurrence of same are addressed (see Chapter 8). Two distinct abiding and fundamental visions of 'freedom for' in Nietzsche's work[2] will be examined initially here, before interrogation of eternal recurrence in spatial terms, together with the issue of reevaluation of values as a spatial movement inviting reconstruction of understandings of freedom. The first 'freedom for' is the unmediated experience of the life will through a universal preconceptual language of music as an expression of the Dionysian counterpole to the Apollonian. This freedom is one of challenging the boundaried self, as a loss of self in the life flow for an experiential ecstasy or rapture that challenges selfconsciousness, an enchantment that Nietzsche drew on from Schopenhauer's movement from the *principium individuationis* that Nietzsche associated with the Apollonian counterpole to the Dionysian. The second 'freedom for' is a monistic vision of the human as giving expression to an accelerated naturalism of the animal, primitive instincts as a manifestation of this version of the life will, most specifically the life will in its subservience to the will to power. This vision follows Nietzsche's propensity for monism, where soul is treated as part of bodily experience, and the human is not a dualistic counterpole to the animal but rather as needing animalistic expression of its instincts.

The throne of the will to power is not merely paved with diametric spatial steps; the throne is carved *into* the steps as diametric space, it *is* the steps, as a sterile ascent. Schiller (1795–1796) distinguishes the naive poet who *is* nature from the sentimental poet who seeks nature; Nietzsche's self-proclamation in Dionysian terms is tantamount to a statement that he is or at least expresses diametric space, as a naive creator in Schillerian terms and yet he also clearly seeks diametric space and is thus a sentimental creator additionally in Schillerian terms. Yet these naive and sentimental vantage points are still a confined ambit, a reduction of expression of life to diametric spatial projected realities.

This second vision of the will to power as involving sacrifice through death, of embracing hate and destruction as dimensions of our instincts to support the strong and dismiss the weaker is closely associated with the other key Nietzschean preoccupation as a 'freedom from' – freedom from cultural constructions of good and evil, as a residue of slave resentment of those aristocratic and with power.

Common threads between both Nietzschean visions of a 'freedom for', are, at least superficially, a concern to give expression to the Dionysian myth and entwined with this, a view of this as the prime expression of a will to life, although the second vision subsumes the will to life as a tool, as a means to the goal of the will to power that gains precedence. The second vision of 'freedom for' is a firm, all pervasive descriptive account of the colonising of experience and the world by diametric spatial projections. The first vision is more enigmatic and can be interpreted as swaying between a fundamental monism as fusion with the unmediated life will in music and a possible concentric spatial relational state as an opened boundary relative to the Apollonian *principium individuationis*. The Nietzschean critique of 'freedom from' is itself thoroughly embedded in diametric spatial projections and assumptions, involving a shifting network of moving from one set of diametric relations to others, in a system without substantive progression beyond this state of relation.

These two 'freedom for' visions offer different implications for the individual. In the first, early Nietzschean vision of the individual fusing with the river of the will to life, this involves a decentring of experience from the ego of the *principium individuationis*. [3] This is a loss of a sense of selfconscious self into a prior overwhelming mode of experience, as an overpowering monism. The second is of the individual subsumed by the will to power force, him or herself exerting a subjective will to power but only secondarily against the background of a prior overpowering will to power background. This vision as will to power is tantamount to systems of diametric spaces subsuming the individual and colonising experience. Yet there is also in Nietzsche's 'freedom from', from the good and evil prescriptions of conventional morality and arguably from habits of perception, a potential opening for a third different kind of 'freedom for'.

Beyond reevaluation of values to restructuring habits of emotion and experience: an emergent vision of 'freedom for'

Exploring the silent spaces lurking within the crevices of Nietzsche's thought, there is a third experiential vision of 'freedom for' hounding at least the edges of Nietzsche's thought in latent spatial modes. This vision incorporates a number of elements as basic concepts of Nietzsche's later thought, including an attempt by Nietzsche to restructure a triumvirate of diametric oppositions – good–evil in the transvaluation of values, pleasure–pain and for–against. These include his attempt to engage in a transvaluation of values, to challenge the traditional Platonic good, leading to free spirits beyond good and evil. This is a vision not only of a shift in values, but also a shift as a *restructuring of habits of emotions and experience*. Allied with this is his proposed mode of selfovercoming and his conception of eternal recurrence. The questions Nietzsche asks are arguably more pertinent than the attempts he makes to answer these questions here for this cluster of thoughts in his later works.

It is not being argued that this third version of 'freedom for' in Nietzsche is a fully fledged coherent framework in his work; rather that it requires understanding in spatial-phenomenological terms to apprehend its firm limitations, the importance of its ambition and to advance some of these key questions of Nietzsche, albeit in a different conceptual and experiential direction from that which he envisaged, namely, in a direction of *inclusion* of the other as part of concentric structured spatial experience. Moreover, much of Nietzsche's concerns arguably pave the way for a preoccupation with both overcoming diametric structured experience and engaging with at least aspects of concentric spatial experience. Where can there be a sweep of air through the locked rooms of diametric space?

Nietzsche challenges the good–evil diametric opposition and is aware of the need to seek a more fundamental understanding. This he locates in a will to power, 'what the people believe to be good and evil betrays to me an ancient will to power' (Z: 136), 'much that seemed good to one people seemed shame and disgrace to another … a table of values hangs over every people … it is the voice of its will to power' (Z: 84). Nietzsche transforms the diametric opposition of good–evil into a diametric oppositional space of will to power. He recognises the Buddhist notion that good and evil are both fetters (GM: 96),[4] at times treating this, albeit *en passant*, as implicating a prior domain of love: 'What is done out of love always takes place beyond good and evil' (BGE: 52). Yet love itself is embedded with hate, 'learn to *despise* when we love' (BGE: 88); this love–hate interplay itself presupposes a power relation. There is little doubt that central features of Nietzsche's thought finds diametric space *simpliciter* somewhat oppressive, even as he lurches from one variant of it to the next, closed within a series of substitutions that do not efface this fundamental dimension of the diametric.

A central feature of Nietzsche's thought, nevertheless, is his propensity to treat monism as the root of some contexts of diametric dualism, where 'good' is derivative from a prior evil and violence and 'good actions are sublimated evil actions' (HH: 75), asking: 'How much blood and cruelty is the foundation of all "good things"?' (GM: 38). Nietzsche seeks to overcome the good–evil opposition through treating the good as derivative, as a sublimation of the evil, 'to admit the possibility of the craving for cruelty not necessarily having become really extinct: it only requires, in view of the fact that pain hurts more nowadays, a certain sublimation and subtilisation' (GM: 43). For Nietzsche, 'the categorical imperative reeks of cruelty', where 'cruelty constituted the great joy and delight of ancient man' (GM: 41). Thus, the strategic response of Nietzsche to the diametric opposition between good and evil is to seek to overcome it, not through a radical restructuring as transformation but to compress this opposition into the Procrustean bed of a monism, of a monistic reduction of good to evil.

The monism of reducing the good–evil opposition to deriving from a fundamental cruelty as evil combines with a further monistic reduction in Nietzsche, namely, the monism of reducing the pain–pleasure opposition to pain as suffering. The apparent primacy of pleasure as joy in Nietzsche's equation of 'will to life, and joy' (HH: 152) still rests of the subordination of will to life to will to power, where joy becomes a celebration of cruelty. Historically, 'even in great *punishment* there is so much which is festive' (GM: 44) as an end of itself, observing 'the continually growing spiritualisation and deification of cruelty, which pervades the whole history of the higher civilisation' (GM: 42). Nietzsche continues:

> [I]t is well to remember the times when men judged on converse principles because they could not dispense with the infliction of suffering, and saw therein a magic of the first order, a veritable bait of seduction to life. (GM: 43)

Suffering is treated as an end of itself and life beholden to this as a means. The fundamental source for derivation, whether for a will to life or power is suffering, 'as deeply as man looks into life, so deeply does he look also into suffering' (Z: 177), with Dionysus as a 'god' who 'suffers' (EH: 75) as the epitome of life and power.[5]

Pleasure as happiness is ultimately subverted by the monistic gravitational pull of the will to power bringing 'The happiness involved in the "smallest superiority"' (GM: 98); the pain–pleasure opposition is derivative from a prior will to power that privileges the infliction of pain as exertion of power. Pain–pleasure thus succumbs again to a monism where pain triumphs.

Wellbeing is subordinate to suffering, as pleasure is to pain: 'Well-being, as you understand it – is certainly not a goal; it seems to us an *end*; a condition which at once renders man ludicrous and contemptible – and makes his destruction *desirable*! The discipline of suffering, of *great* suffering' (BGE: 93). Nietzsche is launching an assault here on an experiential mode of resting in need of protection on the frail vessel, in risk-free retreat against the background storms of life. The experiential slumber of diametric spatial closure to stimuli is being trenchantly assailed here.

His attack is at one with that on a fear of freedom as a closure in wellbeing. It is through a fundamental mode of openness to the background vast expanse of stimuli, the ocean and storms of Schopenhauer[6] that Nietzsche's realm of great suffering arises; it is a basic engagement with what he previously termed original pain, with a mode of expansion that brings with it a suffering, as a dimension of an expansive mode of living in experience. His concern is to challenge flattened notions of comfort and security underpinning some conceptions of wellbeing, while he quests for an experiential intensity connected with risk and danger of destruction of self, 'the devotion of the greatest is to encounter risk and danger and to play dice for death' (Z: 138), with death as a dimension of the will to power.

The pain of suffering is elsewhere expressed by Nietzsche as linked with a sadism, a pleasure or 'happiness' in the suffering of others. It is a suffering envisaged in diametric mirror image inversion terms as being a compensatory process:

> Because the *infliction* of suffering produces the highest degree of happiness, because the injured party will get in exchange for his loss (including his vexation at his loss) and extraordinary counterpleasure: the *infliction* of suffering – a real feast. (GM: 41)

This is strongly resonant with the diametric mirror image atonement found in the sacrificial rites of Dionysian feasts as described by Kerenyi, although Kerenyi stresses the ambivalence of the emotions involved rather than simple happiness.[7]

Kerenyi describes 'the great Dionysian sacrifice, where the sacrificial animal represented a suffering, dismembered god' (1976: 116). Again this is a diametric mirror image function of compensatory atonement. This offers a conceptual backdrop to Nietzsche's account of the will to power as needing death: '[A] will and way to a greater power … is always realised at the expense of innumerable smaller powers. The magnitude of a "progress" is gauged by the greatness of the sacrifice that it requires: humanity as a mass sacrificed to the prosperity of one stronger species of Man – that *would* be a progress' (GM: 51). The primacy of pain as sacrifice is again asserted, here in an abhorrently fascistic fashion. Interfusing life and death: 'Loving and perishing: these have gone together from eternity. Will to love: that means to be willing to die, too' (Z: 145), sacrifice and pain again hold primacy in life, as 'there must be bitter dying in your life, you creators!' (Z: 111).

Nietzsche offers a requiem for constructs of good and bad, but in doing so he resurrects the very diametric space on which good and bad is founded. Nietzsche perceives the limitations of the diametric oppositions, good–evil, pleasure–pain and seeks to overcome them for a purportedly more fundamental level of reality and experience. This is a vital task; however, Nietzsche's response to this offers an ultimately sterile movement from diametric space to monism – a monism of reducing good–bad to cruelty and pleasure–pain to suffering. Far from transcending diametric space, he falls into a vacuum of a flat monism in experiential and conceptual terms. Yet this monism resides ultimately for Nietzsche in the will to power, which is itself a diametric spatial oppositional movement. Thus, the extent of Nietzsche's thwarted life pulse is a movement as staggering between diametric space and monism and back from monism to diametric space, as his own version of a flattened eternal recurrence. This movement is not so much one of a *fort–da*, disappearance and return process; it is rather an omnivorous ubiquity of simultaneously operating structures in the mutual (somewhat dynamic) interplay between diametric space and monism.

Nietzsche's attempt to render relative all historical conceptions of good and evil is part of an agenda not only to deconstruct traditional moral values but also to reevaluate the hierarchy of values. Yet this is only a partly completed conceptual agenda and, at that, a displacement of diametric spatial oppositions between good and evil into prior diametric spaces, namely, those between master and slave, aristocrat and plebeian. The key aspect lacking in Nietzsche is the wider ambition, implicit at times in his work, to *reconstruct primordial habits of experience*. Whereas in places he thinks of animal instincts as being set in stone for humans, there is a recognition that the key primordial habit of responding to pleasure and pain is not necessarily one that can sustain a clear diametric opposition between pleasure and pain, so that both can become mutually infused and parasitic each on the other. While Nietzsche is firmly against an ascetic or other religious forms of seeking to transcend these pleasures and sufferings, whether through abstraction, sublimation or other strategies that are tantamount to Freudian repression, it is clear that suffering is central to fundamental experience for Nietzsche and there are promissory notes for a reconstruction of the relation between pleasure and pain in human experience.

While Nietzsche is launching an assault on *habits as values*, where it is 'a sheer matter of habit they were praised as good' (GM: 10), it needs to be foregrounded that he is also seeking to uproot *habits of emotion and experience*. [8] Even the will to power is understood by Nietzsche in experiential terms in terms of affect, 'the will to power is the primitive form of affect, that all other affects are only developments of it' (WP: 366).

Much of later Nietzsche's work is also strongly preoccupied with an experiential shift, a shift in habits of primordial experience as part of 'a transvaluation of values' (BGE: 70). A key search of his, as part of a third emergent version of 'freedom for' is for 'a new habit, that of understanding, non-loving, non-hating' (HH: 76). While this may offer Buddhist resonances as a link to primitive habits of feeling to be transformed beyond pleasure and pain, it would, if so, not be new. Moreover, Nietzsche rejects 'heart-softening, under the spell of which Europe seems to be threatened with a new Buddhism', while dissecting 'the morality of mutual sympathy' (BGE: 69) along the lines of his previous criticisms of compassion. Yet, even here in the quest for a restructuring of modes of experience, Nietzsche is only seeking a new 'habit' rather than seeking a very malleability to the habitual itself in experience of the present moment. Any restructuring is a replacement of habits, one with another, rather than a dissolution of the habitual as structures underpinning experience. Moreover, he does not address here the *diametric spatial habit* that is seated throughout his accounts of fundamental experience and thought.

Nietzsche spends much time subduing asceticism as a life strategy that subdues itself, as distinct from treating it as an interim approach to unsettle habits of experience. It is not a matter of battering holes into the borders of diametric space; bullets of the mind will not pierce its contours. It is vulnerable not to force but to vulnerability, to the sweeping waves of the moment that can dissolve its walls. This empire of thought becomes empty in the moment.

A later Nietzschean preoccupation is with selfconscious experience as 'self-reflection' and differs starkly from the terrains of preconscious experience, and loss of self in the fusion of a unity with Dionysian music: 'Revaluation of all values: that is my formula for the highest act of self-reflection on the part of humanity' (EH: 88). His earlier concern is with a *shift in modes of experience* not simply modes of selfconscious values, an earlier concern that requires revitalisation in this context.

Elsewhere he seeks to challenge an experiential habit expressed in diametric terms, when questing for a 'free spirit … No longer chained down by hatred and love, one lives without Yes without No' (HH: 8) – a freedom beyond diametric spatial-relational oppositions. Extolling a without 'For or Against' (HH: 9), he associates feeling with habit, 'the power of ancient habits of feeling' (HH: 24), while linking feeling to a power dimension. The argument here for current purposes is that these spaces of feeling are primordial but it is not a claim that they are ancient, while accepting a power dimension in them (HH: 24). Nietzsche treats these feelings as pleasure and pain, 'a more primitive form of the world of emotions, in which everything still lies locked in a mighty unity, which afterwards branches off and develops itself in organic processes … as a kind of instinctive life … as a primary form of life?' (BGE: 27). Nietzsche offers a significant acknowledgment of a quasi-language associated with emotions, 'systems of morals are only a sign-language of the emotions' (BGE: 57). If 'the anthropological engine for the birth of human language is the expression of the fundamental passions' for Rousseau (Quintili 2016: 39), this engine for the birth of human morals is fundamental passions for Nietzsche.

Morals derive from emotions and experience, thus a shift in experiential habits can bring a transformation of values. Nothing less than a restructuring of habits of experience, including emotions, is needed.

Nietzsche's conception of a free spirit is in terms of freedom from, 'released himself from tradition, be it successfully or unsuccessfully' (HH: 140). Interpreting Nietzsche's accounts of free spirits against the backdrop of his call for a shift in experiential habits and in primitive emotional habits, free spirits are not simply engaged in a process of liberation from thought conditioning, but also from *experiential habits, including habitual structures of experience*. Such habits are those inculcated through environmental conditioning, such as conditioned pleasure–pain responses, 'a free spirit if he thinks otherwise than would be expected, based on his origin, environment, class, and position, or based on prevailing contemporary views' (HH: 139).[9] Nietzsche offers some perspective on habits of thought in philosophy that he is challenging. Reflecting on reasoning processes, he offers this panoramic view in terms of oppositions and sublimations:

> In almost all respects, philosophical problems today are formulated as they were two thousand years ago: how can something arise from its opposite – for example, reason from unreason, sensation from the lifeless, logic from the illogical, disinterested contemplation from coveted desire, altruism from egoism, truth from error ? Until now, metaphysical philosophy has overcome this difficulty by denying the origin of one from the other, and by assuming for the more highly valued things some miraculous origin, directly out of the heart and essence of the 'thing in itself'. Historical philosophy ... has determined in isolated cases...that they are not opposites ... there exists, strictly considered, neither a selfless act nor a completely disinterested observation: both are merely sublimations. (HH: 13)

A preoccupation here again is with patterns of dualism to be shattered in some way. Nietzsche's words in his notes on eternal return from August 1881, cited by Heidegger, include 'Pointers Towards a New Life' (Vol. II: 80) and 'Projection of a New Way to Live' (Vol. II: 78). These illustrate not only that the reevaluation of values is fundamentally a search not simply for values for a life principle, but also that this is an experiential quest for new modes of lived experience as life-giving experience.

Eternal return for Nietzsche invites 'the possibility of defining and ordering anew individual human beings in their affects' (number 118), cited by Heidegger (Vol. II: 130). Connecting this with the reevaluation of values, the primary task is an *experiential* restructuring, a recalibration of the spatial modes of primordial experience, an experience projected into values. However, Heidegger (Vol. III: 15) emphasises value and valuation rather than experience in understanding Nietzsche on this theme.

For Nietzsche, morality is not a sealed compartment. It relies fundamentally on external sources for its constituting force and relation. These external circumstances are social conditions of history. They are also resting on experiences; morals are emanating from experience and not handed and hardened down as some eternal truth. Nietzsche did not take the further step of interrogating the structural regularities of these experiences, namely, spatial-structural dimensions of diametric space and beyond.

A spatial-phenomenological tenet is that space is the fabric of experience. On the malleability of space-shaping experience, the potential for malleability of values rests; conditioning forces for values derive from projections of fundamental spatial experience for 'minds strong and original enough to initiate opposite estimations of value, to transvalue and invert "eternal valuations"' (BGE: 69). Nietzsche's transvaluation could simply be reduced here to a contrarian manifesto of opposing and inverting as a diametric spatial projection. This reduction is supported also by his exhortation to 'putting the vivisector's knife to the breast of the *very virtues of their age*' (BGE: 83), typically, a knife that turns into a mirror to bring inverted symmetry as direct reversal of values, including the reversal of the Platonic privileging of the supersensuous realm. This is again a diametric spatial projection of splitting, as assumed separation. Yet a more subtle implication is also possible – that values are based on experiences and transvaluation is based on a restructuring of our basic experiences, our experiential habits. A spatial-phenomenological reading here of Nietzsche would then call into question further experiential possibilities and foundations beyond the hard enamel of diametric spatial boundaries biting into experience. This invites a wider and primordial spatial questioning for experience and experiential transformation in concentric spatial terms.

If values are contingent on emotions and hence experiences, then a shift in values can be developed through a shift in experiences. A shift in values without a transformation in experience is arguably a somewhat redundant process, 'the holy pretext of "improving" humanity recognized as a ruse to drain dry life itself and make it anaemic. Morality as vampirism' (EH: 95). He does not seek a transvaluation as abstraction, divested from experience and emotion, as a desiccation of life. The problem with Nietzsche is that the experiential shift sought is one beset by diametric space, in diametric spatial terms for experience rather than wider experiential modes of transformation. Nietzsche's third vision of a 'freedom for' is an emergent one, halfborn in his work, with echoes of the Dionysian from BT in particular regarding an opening of boundaries and to engage with a level of original pain as a deep suffering, although not simply a diametric spatial splitting.

For Bataille, 'Nietzsche's weakness' is that 'he criticizes from the standpoint of a moving value, whose origin and end he – obviously – doesn't grasp' (1945: 96). Nietzsche at times seeks to replace values through reversal. However, from another vantage point his concern is a phenomenological one, he seeks a shift in the direction of our experiences, our capacity for experience. It is this shift to experiential habits that a quest for a primordial spatial discourse speaks to.

Nietzsche's selfovercoming is a relation between self and other that is an assumed separation on stilts: 'You look up when you desire to be exalted. And I look down, because I am exalted' (Z: 171) (Prelude to Part Three), as up–down mirror image: 'Life wants to raise itself on high with pillars and steps' (Z: 125). Diametric spatial oppositions of high–low are projected onto life as part of turn to power. He seeks 'the Superman. Man is something that should be overcome' (Z: 41).

As with the mere displacement of diametric spatial relations from the good–evil mirror image to the master–slave inversion, Nietzsche's other attempted solution for his 'freedom for' problem of selfovercoming falls again into this ditch of diametric space with his mirror image higher–lower hierarchy in a conception of subjectivity as the overman. This diametric spatial mirror image between the strong and the weak buttresses his will to power framework so that the entire conception of the overman is governed by a diametric spatial oppositional movement. While it is tempting to characterise Nietzsche as a methodological one-trick pony in his repetition of shifts from and between diametric spaces, another interpretation is to seek to refresh the earlier vision of Nietzsche's 'freedom for', his experiential restructuring of the *principium individuationis* in Dionysian music, as a recentring of experience that is pivotal to at least a direction towards growth in human experience,[10] if not an exaggerated, objectionable overman or superman. For current purposes, the two visions of 'freedom for' in Nietzsche are being reinterpreted so as to acknowledge the descriptively accurate destructive vision of diametric space in his latter vision of 'freedom for', while seeking to replace this will to power vision of 'freedom for' with a variant of his first vision of experiential expansion – his excess on the Dionysian, his experiential projection that was an added layer on the Dionysian, a layer than can itself be sustained with a vitality, as a *sui generis*, while excising the very Dionysian flesh around which it wrapped itself.

His selfovercoming can be seen as a mode of response to the fundamental existential dilemma he observed in BT, regarding overcoming the *principium individuationis* to engage with the background storms of life stimuli. Yet his later response of selfovercoming is more one of seeking to gain dominion over the storms through a larger stronger boat, imposing itself on the background ocean as an impregnable self-creating force.

Primarily as a mode of relation of self to him or herself,[11] selfovercoming is a variant of the experiential restructuring already ached for in overcoming the *principium individuationis* of BT. Yet, whereas the experiential restructuring in the loosening from the boundaried Apollonian mode was an opening to a relation ultimately of monism with the background stormy sea of stimuli, as an annihilation of self – and a challenge to the more diametric boundaried state of the Apollonian – the later Nietzschean attempt to restructure experience operates firmly *within* a diametric spatial mode, a mirror image hierarchy. This is scarcely an advance on the earlier, Schopenhauer-inspired, mode of experiential opening and restructuring.

If the earlier mode of opening in the overcoming of the *principium individuationis* offers an affinity with an Eastern quest to go beyond the ego, in the transcending of the veil of *maya*, the later Nietzschean solution of self-overcoming rushes in a diametrically opposing direction, of acceleration of ego, of ego on steroids, all the while that the dominion of diametric space becomes entrenched in this later version of overcoming as selfovercoming: 'My concept of Dionysian became the highest deed here; measured against it, all the rest of human action appears poor and limited' (EH: 71). Again a diametric spatial hierarchy of high and low is beckoned by Nietzsche.

Nietzsche perceives the need to move from diametric oppositions (such as good–bad, pleasure–pain, for–against) though not in *spatial* terms. He moves in the direction of further compression into monism (cruelty, suffering), and does not seek the contrary direction of expansion – such as expansion into concentric space. Nevertheless, he does in BT conceive of an opening, a loosening as some kind of expansive process in a restructuring of experience through a prerepresentative apprehension of music. Moreover, he explicitly conceptualises in terms of a condensing process in the Apollonian, 'condensed into images' (BT: 52), tantamount to a tightening of boundaries as part of a diametric spatial process; *this invites contemplation of the reverse direction from condensing, from compression to concentric expansion as opening.*

As part of a wider experiential structuring for humanity, later Nietzsche does *not* seek to invoke the radical restructuring of experience he envisages for Dionysian rapture in the pre-image-based kind of experience of music he extols in BT. The ambition of this experience is simply as an end of itself, an enchantment that is not be construed in sheer instrumental terms. Its reduction to a purpose, existential or otherwise would not only reduce its experiential intensity for Nietzsche, it would itself be a chimeric goal. Yet this is the first attempt at what Nietzsche would later quest for with regard to a self-overcoming – the Dionysian overcoming of the boundaried self of the Apollonian in experience is a kind of selfovercoming, a movement within the self into a different precognitive experiential site.

While this locus of experience may ultimately lack a coherent concentric spatial understanding in Nietzsche and be rendered rather in monistic terms of fusion with a will to life, echoing Schopenhauer's monism here, this momentary experiential opening, whether as an eruption or otherwise, offers a domain of relevant human experience where pleasure and pain are in some way fused or in assumed connection. As Parkes highlights: '[The] Heraclitean idea of the mutual interdependence of such opposites as pleasure and pain would remain a feature of Nietzsche's philosophical psychology throughout its development' (1994: 35). A site for experience is uncovered that is not one where pleasure and pain are spliced from one another. The enchantment of this experiential opening can be interpreted as a dimension prior to a diametric split between pleasure and pain, a split that is the basis for environmental conditioning through pain and pleasure, positive and negative reinforcement going back to Lycurgus, Helvétius and Bentham, as antecedents of Skinner's behavioural psychology.

Whereas Nietzsche rejects the contents of where 'the saint and ascetic invented a new category of life stimuli' (HH: 99), it is arguable that his pervasive search is for new categories of life stimuli, to go prior to fundamental habits of feeling such as pleasure–pain and of thought as good–evil. His later response to this quest is for the will to power as the overarching category of life stimuli. The proposed primordial spatial discourse of concentric and diametric spaces of relation in relation are not a recourse to a static category or schema structure or set of structures. There is a loss of *élan vital* in any mere categories. The spaces are more dynamic, as directional movements, than mere categories or schemata. Nevertheless, they do pertain to the domain of relevance of uncovering life stimuli. This quest is to go beyond the experiential torpor of the medium of diametric space. The dry season of diametric space is an ossification of experiential possibility, as a loss of the moisture of expanded reception of life stimuli through concentric space.

This conceptual movement between diametric space (pleasure–pain, good–bad) and monism (suffering, cruelty), and back, is at least a movement. It constitutes an animation in primordial spatial terms. It is a repetitive movement within itself – from diametric dualistic oppositions of pleasure–pain, good–bad to respective related monisms of suffering and cruelty. These monisms are themselves drawn from the will to power, which is a diametric oppositional space of dualistic mirror image reversals and assumed separation. This repetitive movement operates not only within these aspects of later Nietzsche's thought but also across his oeuvre. The overcoming of the *principium individuationis* through experience of Dionysian music is itself a movement from the diametric space of the Apollonian as separation to the fused monism of the experience of prerepresentative music – in the passage from boat to background ocean and storms. Foreground–background interaction as a primordial spatial domain of relevance is the terrain of this movement.

Yet the diametric space–monism movement of Nietzsche is a highly limited one in primordial spatial terms. Although significant as a movement in basic concepts, across foundational assumption structures of understanding in Western thought, it is nevertheless a movement more akin to that of a fly scratching its back than of a bird's wings soaring through the air for the pure air that Zarathustra seeks. From diametric space to monism and back is a somewhat colourless movement in thought and experience, lacking a fundamental light of opening. It is a life movement as impulse rather than pulse, rather than a movement of space as the pulse of breath. The consistency, sheer repetition and hiddenness of Nietzsche's governing spatial movement marks it out as being quite compulsive in its projection. A strength of Nietzsche's work is the directness with which he engages concepts revealing this primordial spatial discourse. He has entered a fundamental spatial domain to partly articulate a spatial protolanguage, though unaware of the extent to which he is shaped by its contours, conceptually and experientially.

It is tempting to characterise diametric space and monism as the systole and diastole of Nietzsche's thought. However, the movement falls short of this. The diametric space–monism trajectories provide some movement of animation as an expression of a life force. Nietzsche conquers the domain of impulse within this movement but not the space of the pulse of breath.[12]

Concentric space offers a mode of shifting from the habitual, of a movement to go beyond and also restructure diametric spatial habits of experience, feeling and thought. Whereas Nietzsche's scope was to interrogate the habits of life, feeling and thought, his vision of change for these habits was ultimately a violent one of change by force; in contrast, a concentric dissolving of habits, while also engaging with the extremes of experience and feeling, as well as the foundations of understanding, is a different direction of change – a more fluid transformative process. Structures of experience are not random but they are not simply pregiven, set like a mould in concrete. Rather there is a scope for bounded expansions for experience and following from this in the experiential projections that serve as frames for thought, i.e., the diametric and concentric spatial projections underpinning much of experience including concerns with unifying processes for experience. Concentric space offers an acceleration of experiential space, moving it from pre-set, embedded patterns but not in a simply random or completely open-ended way. This acceleration of experiential space upends habits of experience, feeling and thought.

Concentric space summons an impotence that is a thread itself through the will to power, to wrap itself around and through the will to power as diametric space; the very *space* of the diametric devours the diametric. Space is the very mutiny for diametric space, it writhes out of its grasp and control, as space is never fully at home in the diametric shell that seeks to seal it and seal upon it. Just as air must leave the body, as the breath is never fully cast in the chamber of the body.

Diametric space is no sheer disarray, even in its movement of foundations from a monistic fusion or reduction. It serves as a barrier to connection, a halt on expansion. It operates as a confined space for reverse relations, a stilted set of power relations, like an hourglass waiting to be turned over; and yet when doing so, in the very reversal, retaining its own power as the epitome of its own function. Yet against the background of concentric space, the hourglass of diametric space operates a fragile power, although not a false one.

Notes

1 Parkes emphasises this plurality of manifestations, including where Dionysus is associated with the tree god presiding over the ripening of fruit (1994: 176), with a capacity 'to dissolve the boundaries between the human and animal realms

completely' (1994: 214), 'a Dionysian multiplication of perspectives and affects' (1994: 235) as 'god of many forms' (1994: 340), including wine, intoxication, madness and the dance. Together with Zarathustra's three transformations of the spirit, into a camel, lion and finally a child, in the Dionysus of Zarathustra, resides the wisdom of the serpent and pride of the lion, panther and eagle (1994: 361).

2 Parkes (1994: 318) cites Nietzsche's GM 2:16: 'All instincts that do not discharge themselves toward the outside *turn inward* … [as] the *internalization* of the human being … what later came to be called the "soul". This entire inner world, originally, as thin as if it were stretched between two membranes, extended and expanded and acquired depth, breadth, and height in proportion as outward discharge was *inhibited*.' This could be construed as an expansion from the closed diametric space towards concentric space, as a 'put in' positivist process. A contrasting position is that these spaces, as life dimensions, pre-existed human experience as spatial-structural preconditions for life.

3 See also the debate between Parkes and Davis (Davis, 2015; Parkes 2015, 2015a) on conceptions of the ego in Nietzsche's work.

4 As Parkes highlights, Nietzsche's ambivalence to Buddhism mirrors his conflicting attitudes to Schopenhauer's work through which much of his Buddhist knowledge was mediated (1991: 14).

5 Martin emphasises that Nietzsche may also have been influenced by the Four Noble Truths of Buddhism – that there is suffering, that suffering has a cause, that this cause can be eliminated and there is a path or way through which to do this (1991: 99). Nietzsche appears to treat suffering as a monistic source prior to pleasure and pain. However, Hulin observes that: '[T]he Buddha is unrecognizable in the role of the Asiatic Epicurus which Nietzsche would like to have him play' (1991: 72), while Sprung concludes that: 'Nietzsche's repudiation of Buddhism and Hinduism as "life-denying" is hardly adequate to the Indian conception' (1991: 89). Influences of Buddhist and Daoist traditions on Nietzsche include, for Parkes, 'the themes of the ego as an utterly fictional construct, the radical multiplicity of the "I", and the Dionysian dissolution of the boundaries of the self – all of which find their fullest and most powerful expression in Zarathustra' (1991a: 195–196).

6 Although Schopenhauer's thought is largely rejected in this version of Nietzsche's work.

7 Kerenyi describes 'this ambivalence – the intentional killing of the animal accompanied by compassion for it' (1976: 320) in terms tantamount to diametric mirror image spatial reverse symmetry.

8 These concerns are far from the attempt of Clark and Dudrick (2012) to locate a *will to value* in Nietzsche's BGE. As Janaway confirms, any such will to value is not to be found in Nietzsche's texts, published or unpublished and 'must be regarded as a construct of Clark and Dudrick's own' (2012: 18). This is not to disagree with the position of Nietzsche in (BGE: 268) that Clark and Dudrick emphasise: 'A person's valuations reveal something about the structure of his soul.' This process of structural projection requires interrogation in spatial terms, where values are habits of emotion and experience.

9 The other side of the same coin is Garfinkel's (1967) view of the 'cultural dope' as unable to resist cultural conditioning (see also Downes 2003, 2012).

10 Ultimately, it was Jung, with his appreciation of Eastern thought and the concentric structured mandala as the fundamental central archetype, who understood the shift needed for personal growth to be one in what was in rudimentary terms at least, concentric spatial structured terms (Downes 2011, 2012).

11 Although Nietzsche's sensitivity to gender dimensions is lacking through his blatant misogyny (e.g., BGE: 100–105).

12 As seen in Chapter 6, Nietzsche's very conception of spirit is frequently imbued with diametric spatial features of closure and assumed separation. This is in stark contrast with a conception of *spiritus* as breath in a range of traditions (see Downes 2012 on these in concentric spatial terms).

References

Bataille, G., *On Nietzsche.* Trans. B. Boone. London/New York: Continuum, 1945/2004.

Clark, M. and Dudrick, D., *The Soul of Nietzsche's 'Beyond Good and Evil'.* Cambridge: Cambridge University Press, 2012.

Davis, B. W., 'Reply to Graham Parkes: Nietzsche as Zebra: With both Egoistic Antibuddha and Nonegoistic Bodhisattva Stripes', *Journal of Nietzsche Studies*, 2015, *46(1)*: 62–81.

Downes, P., 'The Relevance of Early Heidegger's Radical Conception of Transcendence to Choice, Freedom and Technology', inM. J. Breen and E.Conway (eds.), *Technology & Transcendence.* Dublin: Columba Press, 2003, 160–173.

Downes, P., 'Concentric and Diametric Structures in Yin/Yang and the Mandala Symbol: A New Wave of Eastern Frames for Psychology', *Psychology and Developing Societies*, 2011, 23: 121–153.

Downes, P., *The Primordial Dance: Diametric and Concentric Spaces in the Unconscious World.* Oxford/Bern: Peter Lang, 2012.

Garfinkel, H., *Studies in Ethnomethodology.* Englewood Cliffs, NJ: Prentice Hall, 1967.

Heidegger, M., *Nietzsche*, Vols III and IV. D. F. Krell (ed.), trans. J. Stambaugh, D. F. Krell and F. A. Capuzzi. New York: HarperCollins, 1987.

Heidegger, M., *Nietzsche*, Vols I and II. D. F. Krell (ed.), trans. D. F. Krell. New York: HarperCollins, 1991.

Janaway, C., 'Nietzsche's Psychology as a Refinement of Plato's', *Journal of Nietzsche Studies*, 2014, 45(1): 12–21.

Kerenyi, C., *Dionysus: Archetypal Image of Indestructible Life.* Princeton, NJ: Princeton University Press, 1976.

Parkes, G., 'The Orientation of the Nietzschean Text', in G. Parkes (ed.), *Nietzsche and Asian Thought.* Chicago, IL: University of Chicago Press, 1991, 3–19.

Parkes, G., 'The Early Reception of Nietzsche's Philosophy in Japan', in G. Parkes (ed.), *Nietzsche and Asian Thought.* Chicago, IL: University of Chicago Press, 1991a, 177–199.

Parkes, G., *Composing the Soul: Reaches of Nietzsche's Psychology.* Chicago, IL: University of Chicago Press, 1994.

Parkes, G., 'Open Letter to Bret Davis: Letter on Egoism: Will to Power as Interpretation', *Journal of Nietzsche Studies*, 2015,46(1): 42–61.

Parkes, G., 'Reply to Bret Davis: Zarathustra and Asian Thought: A Few Final Words', *Journal of Nietzsche Studies*, 2015a,*46(1)*: 82–88.

Schiller, F., *On the Naive and Sentimental in Literature.* Trans. H.Wantabe-O'Kelly. Manchester: Carcanet, 1795–6/1981.

Sprung, M., 'Nietzsche's Trans-European Eye', in G. Parkes (ed.), *Nietzsche and Asian Thought.*/ Chicago, IL: University of Chicago Press, 1991.

Chapter 8

Space as movement: eternal recurrence beyond homogenous time

Eternal recurrence as concentric space interacting with the diametric space of will to power

Despite the relatively inchoate exposition – conceptually, if not imagistically – of his underlying intuition of eternal recurrence, a clear and somewhat neglected spatial structure for eternal recurrence is evident in Nietzsche's work. This spatial structure emerges both at the levels of Nietzsche's imagery and concepts regarding his purportedly heaviest, most burdensome thought of 'the greatest weight' (GS: 273). Space need no longer be the neglected sibling of time for understanding of Nietzsche's eternal recurrence. However, in developing this spatial-phenomenological account of eternal recurrence, it is being sought to build on and go beyond Nietzsche's 'doctrine' rather than offer a mere reconstruction.

Bertram treats eternal recurrence as a 'deceptively teasing delusional mystery' (1919/2009: 12), while Kaufmann refers to it as 'this most dubious doctrine', valued by Nietzsche 'so extravagantly' (1975: 323), 'a rigid crudity' (1975: 332). In contrast, Heidegger's emphasises eternal recurrence as Nietzsche's predominant concept, treated as being even more fundamental than will to power. This relies on a foregrounding of temporal assumptions of eternal return as experience of the moment. Not only does a *spatial structure* of eternal return require firmer consideration, a distinct spatial structure is repeatedly conceived by Nietzsche as one of concentric space. The movements of concentric space are pivotal to eternal recurrence.

Heidegger's account of Nietzsche's Zarathustra describes: 'Time's circling in itself, and hence the ever-recurring same for all beings in time, is *the way in which* being as a whole is. It *is* in the way of eternal recurrence. That is how the dwarf guesses the riddle' (Vol. II: 42). Yet Heidegger focuses on the temporal aspect, more than on the spatial aspect of the circular movement.

Concentric circular movement, a concentric expanse *ad infinitum* is centrally postulated by Nietzsche's concept of eternal recurrence, at the very end of WP, where 'the world as circular movement that has already repeated itself infinitely often and plays its game *in infinitum*' (WP: 549). The circular direction is more implicit in EH, where eternal recurrence of same is 'the unconditioned and infinitely reiterated *circulation* of all things' (EH: 65) (emphasis added).

A confluence of intuitions between Schopenhauer and Nietzsche both lead them into the concentric spatial territory of a circle, a ring of eternity. As Schopenhauer states:

> [T]he genuine symbol of nature is universally and everywhere the circle, because it is the schema or form of recurrence; in fact, this is the most general form in nature. She carries it through in everything from the course of the constellations down to the death and rebirth of organic beings. (WWRII: 477/559)

Both the concept of a structure of recurrence and this as a circular structure can be traced directly to roots in Schopenhauer. Heidegger cites the words of the 19-year-old Nietzsche: 'And where is the ring that ultimately encircles him [the human being]? Is it the world? Is it God?' (Vol. II: 11). Heidegger notes that Nietzsche answers this question two decades later with his eternal recurrence of same. In doing so, Nietzsche is again amplifying a fundamental insight of Schopenhauer, although in this case without attributing any influence to him for this key concept in Nietzsche's later work.

A clear contrast, however, between Nietzsche's eternal recurrence and Schopenhauer's circle of recurrence as 'nature's great doctrine of immortality' (WWRII: 477) is that Schopenhauer firmly roots this 'schema' as 'permanent forms' (WWRII: 483), in Platonic ideal forms. Nietzsche's inverted Platonism treats such eternal recurrence in material terms, as the counterpole still locked within the metaphysics of the ideal–real opposition.[1] Concentric and diametric spaces as dynamically interacting structures of recurrence offer a way out of this ideal–real straitjacket.

In GS, eternal recurrence is described as the heaviest burden in number 341, *das Schwergewicht*; Krell (1991) comments in a footnote that: 'Both Nietzsche and Heidegger appear to hear in the word the related term *der Schwerpunkt*, "center of gravity"' (Vol. II: 21). The co-central point of concentric space for infinite expansion of concentric circles can be interpreted as a centre of gravity.

Parkes contrasts the dynamism of Nietzsche's circular movement with that of Platonic spheres: 'One imagines the goal in Plato to be spherical, the consummate form, whereas in Zarathustra eternity is imagined as a ring [of recurrence], a more complex form composed of circles around an empty center' (1994: 241). Concentric space is not static but is a directional movement, a directional movement of expansion into the ripple effect of ever increasing concentric circles. Moreover, concentric spatial movement is a structure not simply a form, where structure is continuous with experiential content, not split from content as in form. The permeable boundaries of concentric space, with strong openness to background, are far from being iron rings.

Concentric space is not only a fundamental concept for Nietzsche's eternal recurrence; it is seeped into his spatial imagery for a concept that is developed fundamentally imagistically and through linguistic imagery.[2] In Zarathustra, eternity is repeatedly described as 'the wedding ring of rings – the ring of Recurrence!' (Z: 247), again invoking concentric imagery of rings within rings. In Zarathustra, the coils of the serpent, wound in rings around the eagle's throat are symbolic of the circle and ring of eternal return, as Heidegger notes (Vol. II: 46) in his analysis of Nietzsche as offering a spatial discourse through 'the palpable presence of sensuous imagery' (Vol. II: 48). The serpent wound around the sun is another key image of eternal recurrence again in concentric structured terms. Zarathustra is replete with concentric imagery and images of circular movement. These also include Nietzsche's wheel as a concentric image for eternal return: 'Everything goes, everything returns; the wheel of existence rolls for ever' (Z: 234), the rolling ball inviting a circular movement, 'the ball There rolls around every Here' (Z: 234), 'the well of eternity' (Z: 288), 'the golden round ring' (Z: 288).

A key question arises: Can eternal recurrence be understood spatially, not only in terms of concentric spatial movements but also in terms of diametric space? This question can be understood at a number of levels, for instance, how can concentric spatial movements be related to Nietzsche's will to power as diametric spatial projections and to the Dionysian as exemplification of diametric spatial structural movements? A further interrogation would require an understanding of concentric and diametric spaces directly as movements pertaining to eternal recurrence, in other words, that diametric space is also in some way embedded within eternal return as a relation to concentric space.

The relationship between eternal recurrence and will to power in primordial spatial terms

Depending on the reference point for comparison, Nietzsche's will to power can be interpreted as the ultimate principle of Nietzsche's work and hence as illustrating his monistic tendency. Yet Heidegger (Vols I and II) challenges a treatment of the will to power as primary in Nietzsche's work, seeking to amplify the importance of eternal recurrence and to locate will to power as embedded within this primary overarching principle. In doing this, Heidegger offers not so much a challenge to a monistic approach of Nietzsche, but rather seeks a common monistic governing principle in Nietzsche. In Vol. III, Heidegger suggests that:

> Both thoughts – will to power and eternal recurrence of the same – say the same and think the same fundamental characteristic of beings as a whole. The thought of eternal recurrence of the same is the inner – but not the retrospective – completion of the thought of the will to power. (Vol. III: 10)

Heidegger affirms the monistic approach of Nietzsche, rather than envisaging will to power and eternal recurrence as distinct, irreducible principles in dynamic or dialectical tension, as part of a wider dualism; albeit as a tripartite structure of time embracing past, future and the present eternal moment, eternal recurrence serves a monistic function as the grounding principle for Nietzsche's thought, on Heidegger's interpretation. The current questioning seeks to incorporate will to power within eternal return, so that there is not a monism for either but a dynamic movement between dual polarities of concentric and diametric spaces.

A scrutiny of concentric space shares with Nietzsche a quest for the primordial and this does not deny the factual accuracy of Nietzsche's accounts of the primordial as will to power in terms of diametric space; however, it does betray the one-sidedness in Nietzsche's quest for the primordial that tears open experiential foundations. Nietzsche accurately perceived one stone within the primordial, the foundation stone of diametric space. However, did he do so at the price of a blind spot towards the primordial interplay and dance this stone engages in, as it bobs on the ocean of concentric space? Eternal recurrence offers a counterpoint to such a view of Nietzsche as lacking a counterpole to will to power as diametric space. Eternal recurrence offers a wider framework than will to power to temper the dim wall of the diametric casting its shadows into the human heart and will.

Time as a circular movement rests on an explication in spatial terms of a circle. Space is far from being a lick of paint over the crevices of the potentially irreconcilable concepts will to power and eternal recurrence, the former as a process of becoming, the latter appearing to invite a more static conception of being. Rather, space is embedded as an explanatory structure central to both. Nietzsche seeks to integrate being and becoming in his eternal return: 'That *everything recurs* is the closest *approximation of a world of becoming to a world of being*' (WP: 330). Space offers such a basis for inclusion of being and becoming, each within the other.

While the Dionysian dimensions of will to power as diametric space have been explored in Chapter 6, there are also strong Dionysian threads in eternal recurrence, as a cycle of life–death rebirth. Nietzsche explicitly links Dionysus and Zarathustra to 'the eternal recurrence of existence … the eternal "yes" to all things' (EH: 73). Dionysus is an archetypal symbol of indestructibility, of death and rebirth, as a core thesis of Kerenyi and this underpins the whole assumption of eternal recurrence. Moreover, Kerenyi's central argument is that the Dionysian myth is one of the indestructibility of life, as a repetition of self. This leaves more than a seed of the Dionysian in Nietzsche's subsequent concerns with eternal recurrence. However, while the Dionysian may be associated with an indestructibility – whether as a life force or will to power, the association of concentric space with a life drive is not to be similarly construed as one of indestructibility. On the contrary, the very concentric structure, even in eternal return, is one that is fragile; it is not a direction of inevitability, even as a life drive, it is vulnerable to being broken into a reduction as diametric space. Concentric space as a movement is a directional possibility, a horizon of movement and not a pregiven reality in the referential world.

A renewed focus is needed on each spatial structure as a directional projection. *Projection is a dynamic return of the same.* A diametric spatial structure is both a positional and directional dimension. As a directional process of projection, the diametric space feeds off itself. Whether as a rectangle, square or circle divided in half, each projective movement in diametric space follows a distinctive trajectory – a linear path where the boundary of the diametric pole serves as a new axis of symmetry for a new mirror image inversion. Diametric spatial directional projection ineluctably occupies a linear space in its movement to recreate itself. In contrast to the hall of mirrors of diametric space, the concentric structure, in pure form as a circle within a circle occupying the same central point, brings a projective directional movement outwards to create further wider circles. Its projective directional movement is in circular expansion to recreate its own structural formation. Expressed in terms of entailments of relative differences between diametric and concentric spaces as dynamic directions, a fourth entailment of the relative differences between diametric and concentric space is that a diametric spatial structural projection moves in a more linear direction and a concentric spatial structural projection expands in a more circular direction (Downes 2012).

A time in which whither becomes whence is held active through a projection of space. A whirling gulf of concentric space spreads far around its circles. The aching space of concentric expansion is not a matter of ascending steep and lofty cliffs; it is a rejection of a linear ascent that does not equally explore the houselessness of descent.

Concentric and diametric spaces are not simply structures but also movements. Concentric spatial and diametric spatial movements involve different directions of movement. A concentric spatial expansion is a circular expansion as an infinite expansion, a diametric spatial movement is a linear movement towards infinite expansion; diametric space is a linear movement through the axis of symmetry as a series of mirror images. This entailment of the relative differences between concentric and diametric expansive spatial movements offers a horizon for understanding Nietzsche's account of the dwarf in Zarathustra: 'All truth is crooked, time itself is a circle' and 'Everything straight lies' (Z: 178). With time as expansion of infinite concentric spaces, this treats the linear movement of diametric space as a kind of illusion, a veil of *maya*, hearkening back to the early Nietzschean quest to overcome the *principium individuationis* through prerepresentational experience in music. A circular outward movement is more inclusive as a more unifying direction, and arguably is more fundamental than a linear direction.[3] *Diametric spatial movement is a linear movement that is one of exclusion of what is outside the diametric space.* The furrows of diametric space leave a sterile track, yet one that retains an animation, a crust of momentum. *Concentric space as infinite expansion of concentric circles is a more inclusive process as it expands to include ever wider structures of concentric space* – and within these structures there is the lived experience of openness to movement of opening of walls of the diametric.

Zarathustra sets up an initial directional opposition, not only in relation to time but also through spatial imagery of a lane and gateway:

> [T]his gateway … has two aspects. Two paths come together here: no one has ever reached their end. This long lane behind us: it goes on for an eternity. And that long lane ahead of us – that is another eternity. They are in opposition to one another, these paths; they abut on one another: and it is here at this gateway that they come together. The name of the gateway is written above it: 'Moment'. (Z: 178)

Zarathustra asks: 'Do you think, dwarf, that these paths would be in eternal opposition?' (Z: 178). The answer of the dwarf is key to this vision and riddle: 'Everything straight lies', murmured the dwarf disdainfully. 'All truth is crooked, time itself is a circle' (Z: 178). In other words, *the temporal opposition between lanes of the past and future are mere linear constructs that derive from a prior circular truth and time*. It is the circular movement that is pivotal. Diametric spatial movement in a linear fashion gives way to concentric spatial movements, through the mediating dimension of the moment, as the gateway that connects not simply past and future, but concentric and diametric spaces as spaces of infinite movement in eternal opposition as contrasting directions.

Heidegger's interpretation of eternal recurrence examines circularity and linearity in subservient terms to time as the basic organising concept, through the apparel of past and future interrelation:

> [I]f both ways extend to eternity, they wind up at the same place; they meet there, they link up and form one uninterrupted highway. What to us looks like two straight avenues taking off in opposite directions is in truth that segment of an enormous circle which is visible to us here and now, while the circle itself perpetually revolves back upon itself. (Vol. II: 42)

Continuing his interpretation of Nietzsche's dwarf in Zarathustra: '[T]he dwarf understands nothing of what Zarathustra means when he says – bewilderingly enough – that the two paths "affront each other" in the gateway … The two avenues, future and past, do not collide at all, but pursue one another' (Vol. II: 56). Yet this mirror image relation between future and past in opposite directions is a displacement from a more fundamental spatio-temporal movement between concentric and diametric space, ones that do collide and affront one another in lived experience of the moment.

Against this spatial-phenomenological backdrop, two contrasting spatial directional movements of concentric circular spatial expansion *ad infinitum* and linear diametric spatial movement *ad infinitum* are the core features of eternal return. These affect the past–future linear time axis but go beyond this version of temporal movement.[4] Eternal return confronts the heavy and weary weight of the portcullis of diametric space, through a shift in the breath of the spatial frames.

Concentric and diametric spaces are far from being simply different directional spaces operating over and through different domains of space. They are thoroughly intertwined, not only in the mutually compensatory function between each space recognised by Lévi-Strauss for its anthropological manifestations in myths, social and physical structures. *Both concentric and diametric space are structural modifications of each other.* They operate in dynamic tension of mutual opposition, for example, through direct contrasts between axes of opening and closure, assumed connection and separation. Mutually chained and entwined, *each space resists the movement of the other.* Nietzsche glimpses this indirectly with his recognition that: 'But all expansion, incorporation, growth means striving against something that resists' (WP: 374) as part of the will to power. The mutual expansions of concentric and diametric spatial movements are eternal re-turnings to same as projected spatial structures, yet *each space thwarts the other's return.*

This resistance between spatial movements is resonant also with Schopenhauer's emphasis on the role of tension. Tension and movement are key tenets of Schopenhauer's understanding, 'everything is in permanent tension and forced movement' as part of 'the blind will appearing as the tendency to life' (WWR II: 359). The contrast with Schopenhauer is that the directional movement is not simply blind but spatially patterned, in both concentric and diametric directional terms. The openness of the interactive tension between these directional pulling spaces invites undecidability, a lack of predetermined outcomes, a distance from teleology as inevitability that could be construed as blind, but it is a movement that is not without directional pattern.

A foreground level of diametric and concentric spaces as positional structures needs to be distinguished from a background level questioning their mutual interactions as directions. This is part of a selfreferential questioning as to whether the background space between concentric and diametric spaces is *itself* a diametric one of splitting or a concentric one of assumed connection? It is not simply a question of a static glue between concentric and diametric spaces but a question of the primordial domain of their interaction.

Concentric and diametric spaces share a common terrain, akin to Nietzsche's gateway, rather than offering each other a great glance of mutual politeness over differing territories. The thwarting of diametric and concentric spaces, each by the other, thereby jeopardises certainty in the eternal return; it invokes a fragility, due to the strife between diametric and concentric spaces, yet still the movement is one of return. The pulse of both movements, as movements and as counter-movements, is one in the directions of return. Directions of return do not mean positions of return; return as contrasting directions of concentric and diametric spatial movements over a common site of interaction coughs up different positions in this cacophonous clash – a clash that may also bring a dance as a dissolution of the diametric into the concentric.

Heidegger's *configuration* question for eternal recurrence is addressed through this spatial structural questioning, through specific spatial relations of concentric and diametric spaces. The *domain* question also asked by Heidegger invites a related questioning in phenomenological terms as to how eternal recurrence relates to lived experience. Heidegger interprets this as through experience of the moment, building on this point in Zarathustra regarding the gateway 'Moment' in the dialogue with the dwarf. Concentric and diametric spaces offer further development of this to describe a protolanguage of space-shaping experience and framing thought, while escaping mere reduction to subjectivism and anthropocentrism as a wider life principle.

Where is the site of overlap between the two infinite movements of concentric spatial expansion as inclusion and the diametric linear expansion as exclusion? Both are entwined conceptually where one is a modification of the other. Moreover, experientially a site of primordial experience mediates their mutual interaction, experience in the moment. Both contrasting directions tear at the heart of human experience, both movements as infinite series frame the horizons of the human breath for experience, as a precondition for experience projected into thought.

Lived experience is the *asymptote* between concentric and diametric spaces, mediating circle and line; the dance of primordial experience mediates the ongoing interactive tension between concentric and diametric spatial movements in their mutual stretching out *ad infinitum*, in contrasting directions held together through the common gateway of experience. The convergent infinite series of diametric spaces dances with and stamps on the divergent infinite expansion of concentric spaces, as two directions entwined in a conflict.

While Taylor treats 'what is being captured' in Nietzsche's eternal recurrence at the end of WP as 'a heightened moment of inspiration' on Nietzsche's part (2007: 245), eternal recurrence within time in lived experience of the moment is of direct relevance for diametric and concentric spaces of experience. Diametric and concentric space offer different kinds of centre of gravity for experience in their respective axes of symmetry; the diametric is a closed wall, the concentric offers an emptying of space at the centre, as a connective patterned space. A shift from reliance solely on diametric structured experience to concentric structured experience brings a shift in the centre of gravity for experience.

The chained vulture of diametric space exerts itself as will to power. As a chain, it enchains and is itself further enchained. Diametric space can be interpreted as a dividing membrane from experience of the direct present moment, its axis of symmetry serves as a line of division between both poles as a wall from the present moment. Concentric space offers a structure of openness to the present moment, where its point of symmetry is one without walls, as a permissive space. Diametric space displaces from experience of the present moment, moving experience into fragmentation as the past and future, with future as mirror image of the past, the unfulfilled threads as the lost contours for and from the past.

On this view, when Nietzsche refers to eternal recurrence as a recurrence of same, sameness is being interpreted as meaning primordial unity, sameness as a direction towards unity rather than a static, flat inert identity. Willing is a directional movement, a movement in space and of space. Zarathustra's 'I shall return eternally to this identical and self-same life' (Z: 237) may at least on a *prima facie* examination imply such a static inert identity, although much rests on the conception of relation between Zarathustra and the human. In contrast to the swift breath of the circling air of concentric space, two vast legs of space are installed in diametric opposition, where everything remains beside in a perpetual mode of side-by-sideness, as if stasis itself could be entrenched into a dynamism.

A flat echoless voice of diametric space nevertheless offers a movement within its sealed space that is more than the collapse into mere monism. Space is not a mere wave beneath an external will to power; space thoroughly saturates and constitutes will to power, through the far from soft murmur of diametric space. Many voiced echoes through concentric space are suppressed into lost pangs, as division in the moment itself, lost as diametric space. Diametric spaces split and close again behind, tearing itself further apart all the while that it summons itself to expand *ad infinitum* in a linear path. This linear pathway movement is driven through the axis of symmetry bringing mirror image expansion.

Concentric space as a fragile space, is not a quenchless space, it can be extinguished. Moreover, diametric space can also be extinguished, not only through being dissolved into concentric space but it can also extinguish itself as a process of self-destruction through the very imposition of its own splitting process on itself.

Diametric space is as a wound to concentric space and a scar emerging from this wound, broken and untrembling. The delegated power of diametric space is a loss of concentric space. Losing a capacity to live in that portion of life around the self, living loses its aroundness to the behemoth of diametric space imposed on experience. A draining of concentric space leads to the vast sands of diametric space.

Linear expansion as the movement of diametric space becomes bereft of momentum and implodes in a reverse linear regression; diametric space divides itself into its self-destruction. The mirror image function operates within diametric space *as a movement*; it offers an *outward* linear expansion *ad infinitum and* a linear *regression* into infinitely smaller spaces of diametric division. The splitting process of movement both *expands and contracts* its domain of deliverance. These opposing directions within diametric spatial movements itself brings the distinction between diametric space as destruction and diametric space as an active movement of mirror image reversals in an outward linear direction. The destruction of splitting and the expansion albeit in a restricted space of mirror image symmetry are both features of diametric space and of diametric spatial movements, *although in diametrically opposing directions themselves*. This reveals the turn to destruction embedded in diametric space, all the while that it unfolds itself in a process of exertion of power over new domains through its expansive linear projection through mirror image symmetry.

Parkes highlights 'the problem of ordering the multiplicity of drives' (1994: 281) is part of the experiential restructuring that is a precondition for a reevaluation of values. He asks 'how to avoid a tedious monarchy of the ego without lapsing into chaos and psychosis' (1994: 368). Parkes continues, highlighting the need for a precognitive resolution rather than a cognitive imposition on drives in experience from a monocentred ego, 'The traditional 'top-down' hierarchy of faculties is reconfigured as a field of drives of varying intensities battling it out among themselves' (1994: 292). *This restructuring is a spatial restructuring* for experience. Concentric space is far from a resiling from the multiplicity and diversity of drives, it is an experiential embracing of these drives in experience (if not action). The horizontal drives have their roots in the archaic past, while the vertical spaces of concentric relational background in its interplay with diametric space offer a vertical directional mode of direct lived experience to transform the horizontal movements. Drives exist not against a blank space background but within an interactive space of experience.

Concentric space offers a background ordering principle for the multiplicity of desires and drives, a spatial ordering principle that offers a directional unity and which distinguishes order from a mere orderliness of abstraction such as Socratic rationalism and Cartesian egoistic thinking selfconsciousness. In doing so, it is an antidote to the narcotic of power, a restructuring of and from the diametric spatial domain of will to power. Yes, this presupposes a power shift between concentric and diametric space in individual experience, yet the concentric spatial direction as movement is not a power as hierarchy but as an expansive life force in the cosmos.

The flow of concentric spatial movements in experience thrives as a background space to dissolve the multiple competing foreground drives into the eternal recurrence of lived experience of the moment. This dissolution is far from inevitable and the turn towards diametric space in the moment, as a spatial and experiential displacement from the moment thwarts the dissolving of the impulses and drives into a wider whole to freshen this wider whole. Concentric space is the spatial receptacle of experience within which the multiplicity of drives is immersed. The lived in spaces entertaining the drives embrace the ripple effect of a concentric spatial ripple of affect.

Foreground–background levels are not a metaphysics as background space is an embedded dimension of a material world that is not some sheer abstraction. The focus is not only *at* foreground and *at* background levels but *between* foreground and background levels. These levels are in mutual interaction, where foreground can be dissolved into the background space.

The experiential movement is not only from diametric space to inhabit concentric space, but it goes further to embrace a dissolving of diametric space, of the thick partition of diametric spatial boundaries into the more transparent porous contours of concentric space. Concentric space takes diametric space in its grasp – the thick partition not only between self and other but also a thick partition dividing experience of the moment.

If diametric space imports a structure of atonement, of compensation through the mirror image reversal – if diametric space proffers a structure of sacrifice, yet it must itself be sacrificed through a wider process, a process of dissolution into concentric space. Concentric space as a sacrifice itself of the diametric structure of sacrifice is not a splitting as dismemberment; it is a different dying as dissolution.

Heidegger asks: 'Is it not the case that the doctrine of return not only can be united with will to power but also constitutes *its sole and proper ground*?' (Vol. II: 153). The argument for eternal return as concentric and diametric spaces can support this suggestion of Heidegger, but only while construing will to power as a narrower feature and limited dimension of eternal recurrence. Yet on another wider view of will to power as tension *between* concentric and diametric spaces, as distinct from the sheer propagation of diametric space, it could be open to interpretation that will to power and eternal recurrence are interchangeable. However, the propagation of concentric and diametric spaces is scarcely to be interpreted as being merely instrumental, as serving a prior goal of power as will. Rather, they are propagated as ends of themselves and, while this goal may place them in mutual tension, the tension does not precede these movements as goals in themselves.

Such a view would require rejection of the narrower view of Nietzsche regarding eternal return as a hammer 'in the hand of the most powerful man' [see Z: II 5a], a view observed by Heidegger (Vol. II: 155) as a key link in Nietzsche between eternal return and will to power. This view firmly limits eternal recurrence to the domain of diametric space. Moreover, Heidegger treats a view of subordinating eternal return to will to power as 'too hasty' (Vol. II: 162), even where eternal return is viewed by Nietzsche as resting on presuppositions. The concentric 'will of the ring' (Z: 332) as a life principle needs to be distinguished from the diametric space of a will to power principle, with both as counterpoles of movements of eternal return.

Eternal recurrence comes to fruition not only in lived experience of the moment. It is this and more. Eternal experience as lived experience of and in the moment would reduce this phenomenon to mere subjectivity rather than acknowledging its wider scope as a cosmological life principle. Moreover, eternal recurrence is not simply within time as subservient to linear time but is rather a primordial precondition for such time. Whereas Nietzsche at times tends to identify the will to power and eternal recurrence, a different interpretation is to treat eternal recurrence as the embodiment of a life principle, including concentric space, so that a power principle of the will to power is not necessarily dominant on a life principle. In other words, the dominion of diametric space in the will to power is not the only possible dominion; concentric space can dissolve diametric space so that life can incorporate power but not be reduced to it. Concentric space offers ample power to subdue the reign of diametric space in experience, though this subjugation is far from an inevitability but is an ongoing struggle in the moment.

If not fully stripped of its Dionysian feathers, Nietzsche's eternal recurrence at least recognises the need for different plumage to soar towards a different mode of experience from the diametric space of will to power. Shaking the extinguished space of the diametric, to render more porous its walls for experience of the trembling moment, the temporal frame for concentric experience *simpliciter* is in direct present experience of the moment. It seeks to shed the derelict momentum of the diametric walls of past-based reactive experience. Encompassing a dissolution process of struggle with diametric space, the directional movement of concentric space is both the present moment lived experience and a futural directional pull.

Space is the bridge between experience and pattern, between lived experience and dynamic structure. Examined in terms of concentric and diametric spaces, a flat domain of 'presence' of these spaces is not being postulated. Three levels can be distinguished.[5] The domain of eternal recurrence as concentric and diametric spaces needs to distinguish i) the level of their interaction as spatial symmetries of unity and inverted symmetry, which is the domain of the primordial, including primordial experience, from ii) the domains in the world and in experience where symmetry is broken, where there are only mere fragments and traces of this primordial spatial interaction. The goal of a unifying direction for experience as primordial experience can be restated as one of engaging with domains of experience pertaining to symmetry, whether symmetry as unity or inverted symmetry – which is *spatialised experience*. Spatialised experience is to be distinguished from a flat experiential monism, a crushed space; experientially, spatialised experience is the site of the awareness of breathing, of the breath as a concentric connective relation to the body in the moment.

These levels i) and ii), still need to recognise iii), a prior background level of dynamic interaction, of a dance and strife between concentric and diametric background directional spaces and not simply foreground positional spaces. Eternal recurrence paves its dynamic paths as movements at the background and foreground levels of these interactions between concentric and diametric spaces. These interacting primordial spaces offer a unity that is at once pattern and goal, purpose and principle, they are together a structure and process, a being and becoming. Whereas the will to life is blind for Schopenhauer, the spatial directional movements of concentric and diametric spaces are not entirely blind but structurally motivated in the clash between their contrasting directions.

There is an elegant simplicity at the heart of a life principle, before it gets torn asunder into fragments of fragments so that not even the limited unity of sorts of diametric space can be sustained. This simplicity is neither one of sheer presence of concentric spaces, nor is it that of mere monism as a limiting condition for the hegemony of one diametric polarity over the other in a mirror image hierarchy.

Life as vitality claims its own space. As a life force or power it is a spatial movement, a movement that claims itself. This life-giving movement is not subjugated by or to power, it encompasses its own power as vitality, as movement; this movement is an end of itself, not a means, not a means to power. The diametric is dissolved into the concentric spatial movement rather than being a means towards the movement of concentric space; similarly, will to power as diametric space is restructured in a dissolving process into being subsumed within the life force of concentric space. This claiming of its own space as both concentric and diametric spatial movements is Nietzsche's eternal recurrence, with the concretising spatial protolanguage also adding the dynamic dimension of interactive tension between both spatial movements over a common terrain, including lived experience. The living spaces of concentric and (in a lesser sense of living) diametric spatial movements strive to preserve themselves and to expand their terrains of relative vitality.

Taylor's carnival inversion as a diametric mirror image space for play: search for a life principle prior to a homogenous space as monism

Eternal recurrence offers a challenge to a flattened, homogenous time. This challenge commingles Nietzschean concerns with those of Charles Taylor in his *magnum opus, A Secular Age*, with Taylor's preoccupation with loss of carnival as draining Western society of a life force or principle, offering a further resonance with Nietzsche's Dionysian thematic. Yet their common temporal concerns require a reorientation in terms of space, for a spatial protolanguage to vivify the flattening of the temporal in experience.

The erasure of carnival is given a particular prominence in Taylor's work. The decline of this space for play as a dimension of a life principle, and consequent change in its function, is treated as a pivotal step in the historical development of what he describes as the homogenous, secular time, underpinning lived conditions of modernity. This is, by no means, the sole strand of Taylor's interplay of a range of dimensions to the historical construction of homogenous, secular time. However, it is a feature inviting further critical scrutiny through explication, not simply in terms of temporality but additionally of *spatiality*.

Nietzsche refers to 'Dionysian drunkenness and mystical self-abandonment', 'Dionysian festivities' bringing 'an effusive transgression of the sexual order' (BT: 24), 'the Dionysian state, with its annihilation of the usual limits and borders of existence' (BT: 46). Whether this close proximity between medieval carnival and Nietzsche's Dionysian expression is intended by Taylor or otherwise, it is not the *mens rea* question but the following one, which is more apposite: is the loss of carnival and festival features of inversion, whether viewed as suppression of the Nietzschean Dionysian counterpole or otherwise, an important contributing factor to a homogenisation of *space* as part of a loss of a life principle?

While Taylor would justifiably baulk at Nietzsche's wholesale rejection of Enlightenment values of egalitarianism, his engagement with Nietzsche's work recognizes the force both of its influence on postmodernist thought and also of its critique of a supposedly repressed state of middle ground existence, associated with humanism, which Nietzsche would view as limiting the heroic, individual dimension to existence. Taylor's accounts of carnival and festival for medieval Europe resonate strongly with Nietzsche's description of Dionysian festivals in BT, invoking 'the eternal truths of the Dionysian and the Apollonian' (BT: 105).

Taylor's preoccupation is with 'the different kinds of lived experience invoked in understanding your life in one way or the other, on what it's like to live as a believer or unbeliever' (2007: 5). This amounts to a phenomenological focus on 'lived conditions' (Taylor 2007: 8), prior to beliefs, which then leads into a thematising of temporality, as one such condition. The Heideggerian resonance to these phenomenological commitments is explicitly acknowledged by Taylor, in his search for 'the usually unspoken, background understanding' (2007: 95), rather than intentional beliefs, as such. Necessary or key conditions for lived experience tend to invite focus on background temporal and spatial conditions, in Heidegger's terms, on a background horizon of understanding. For early Heidegger, these conditions are *structures* of being located in a primordial temporal dimension prior to linear historical time. Taylor has reoriented the lens of concern for religious and other forms of belief away from the cognitive contents of belief as being primary. He has performed an important shift of trajectory from belief to experience, to conditions of experience and aspects of relation, to a kind of existential history, in apprehension of putative dimensions to a loss of transcendence.

The full scope of Taylor's argument need not be rehearsed here. Suffice to point out, for current purposes, that Taylor makes explicit a mode of time that is homogenous and empty and links this with the rise of secularism in Western society, 'this identification of time in cosmic terms makes it an indifferent container of … human and historical events … In that sense, cosmic time is (for us) homogenous and empty' (2007: 58). Taylor's insight has obvious resonance with an argument that space may not simply be homogenous and empty, as a lived condition for certain modes of experience. This invites questioning, as to what extent can a conception of spatial relation also be similarly viewed as a flat, homogenous and empty mode.

Taylor continues:

> Time has become a precious resource, not to be 'wasted'. The result has been the creation of a tight, ordered time environment. This has enveloped us, until it comes to seem like nature ... This 'time frame' deserves, perhaps more than any other facet of modernity, Weber's famous description of a '*stahlhartes Gehäuse*' [iron cage]: It occludes all higher times, makes them even hard to conceive. (2007: 59)

Time frames are connected with space frames; and homogenous time and secularism are supposedly tethered to one another. However, Taylor is focused, not so much on what early Heidegger would prioritise as primordial experience, but rather on a domain of relevance of ordinary experience. Taylor does acknowledge the interrelation between homogenous time and homogenous space, stating that, with the achievement of perspective in painting in the fifteenth century, 'we get objects which are clearly ranged in a single coherent space' and 'the coherence of space has to mean the coherence of time too'(2007: 96). Yet, it is the flattening process of this spatial coherence and homogenisation that requires further explication. The tight ordered domain of diametric space that envelops us has occluded a concentric spatial mode of experience.

Taylor has, in one sense, basically fleshed out some of the sociohistorical dimensions to Heidegger's distinction in *Being and Time* between a linear historical time and a purportedly more authentic mode of primordial temporality, what Heidegger views as a temporal transcendental horizon for the question of being. The Ariadne thread of Taylor's argument is succinctly summarized in his words: '[T]he horizontal flow of secular time ... is another of the great shifts, along with disenchantment, and the eclipse of anti-structure, which have helped to set the conditions for modern secular society' (2007: 59). The dimension inviting further scrutiny, for current purposes, is his claim that the eclipse of anti-structure helped pave the way for the homogenous time of secular, lived experience. The rupturing of anti-structure facilitated the mutation into secular, homogenous time, according to Taylor's thesis.

Taylor describes how carnivals and other festivities in medieval Europe were 'periods in which the ordinary order of things was inverted, or "the world was turned upside down"':

> For a while there was a ludic interval, in which people played out a condition of reversal of the usual order. Boys wore the mitre, or fools were made kings for a day; what was ordinarily revered was mocked, people permitted themselves various forms of licence, not just sexually but also in close-to-violent acts, and the like. (2007: 45–46)

Citing the work of Turner (1969, 1978), Taylor observes:

> These rituals of reversal are in fact very widespread. For instance, in the enthroning ritual of the king in various African societies, the candidate must pass through an ordeal, in which he is reviled, hectored, and even kicked and shoved by his subjects to be. (2007: 48)

Taylor offers a gamut of explanations from commentators regarding this phenomenon. Here the primary interest is in a potential opening, with regard to unexplicated spatial features underlying reversal rituals, such as medieval carnivals.

Diametric spatial inversion of carnival is treated by Taylor as a key mediator against secular, homogenous, flattened time; this also contrasts somewhat with Lévi-Strauss' view based on cross-cultural observations that concentric relation is the mediator for change from diametric relation, usually towards a triadic level of relation.[6] This contrast is not necessarily a contradiction. Diametric inversion is a movement of opening compared to flattened monism, which Taylor suggests was the role of carnivals after the French revolution:

> The epoch of the French Revolution is perhaps the moment in which at one and the same moment anti-structure goes into eclipse ... This emerges most clearly in the attempts of the various revolutionary governments to design festivals which would express and entrench the new society ... But the nature of the enterprise was in a certain sense reversed. That is because the dimension of anti-structure was totally missing. The aim of the exercise was not to open a hiatus in the now reigning code, but to give expression to its spirit and inspire identification with it. (2007: 51)

While this is an interesting historical hypothesis, Derrida's (1978: 42) reservation regarding Foucault's account in *The History of Madness* of the singular classical moment, the deciding gesture for the structure of exclusion as the fundamental structure of historicity, is also to be shared here.[7] Thus, a caveat to Taylor's example of the French Revolution is that it is more an important example, as sample, than as the singular historical model of the eclipse of anti-structure in Western society.

Yet aside from issues of historical causality and influences, the kernel of Taylor's argument is that *a monistic dimension to carnival replaced a diametric one of inversion* – and this change was key to the development of a secular, homogenous time. A monistic mode of time fostered an experiential flattening. Interpreted thus, Lévi-Strauss' view of concentric structures as providing a mediating role can become understood as a further aspect of growth along an opening from monism to diametric spatial opposition to concentric spatial relation and beyond. Allowing for a consistency between Taylor's and Lévi-Strauss' analyses in this fashion, imports a structural temporal dimension of change between these spatial structural modes of relation. Reversing Taylor's historically focused direction of movement from diametric inversion to monism as loss of conditions for experience supporting religious belief, a different directional focus places the direction of movement from monism towards diametric inversion and after to concentric relation, with each prior dimension mediating the one that follows. And this direction of movement is not necessarily identical to linear time, all the while that it commingles with its material events and patterns within linear history.

The centrality of diametric inversion for Taylor's historical movement in the West towards secular time is buttressed by the recognition that the purpose of this inversion was not to destroy the established order but that it acted as a maintenance of, and assumed identification with, this order. The diametric oppositions in social roles were to be reinforced, not challenged:

> The enigma is particularly strong for us moderns, in that the festivals were not putting forward an alternative to the established order, in anything like the sense we understand in modern politics, that is, presenting an antithetical order of things which might replace the prevailing dispensation. The mockery was enframed by an understanding that betters, superiors, virtue, ecclesial charisma, etc. ought to rule. (2007: 46)

Periods of carnival were not so much a caveat to a social contract, as a voracious expression of its implied terms. In medieval Europe, carnival and festival thereby served as nourishment for a diametric structured society of clear oppositions of social role, supported by periodic inverted symmetries.

The key feature of inversion, in carnival and play, is emphasized, by Taylor, in terms of its temporal features and its contribution to a levelling of time into a secularity and homogeneity. Yet developing an understanding of inversion as a mirror image symmetry, of diametric dualistic relation, introduces the issue of space – and transformation of spatial conditions as lived experience.

These diametric structured inverted symmetries, as dimensions of play at a cultural level, can be interpreted as the collective concomitant of the inversions in individuals' play and ritual behaviour, highlighted in Freud's work on obsessional neurosis, in particular. Freud's well-known description, in *Beyond the Pleasure Principle*, of a boy 'greatly attached to his mother', who 'had an occasional disturbing habit of taking any small objects he could get hold of and throwing them away from him into a corner, under the bed, and so on' (1920: 14), is not without criticism (see, for example, Derrida 1987: 298 on the selectivity of Freud in his descriptive process). In Freud's account:

> I eventually realized that it was a game and that the only use he made of any of his toys was to play 'gone' with them. One day I made an observation which confirmed my view. The child had a wooden reel with a piece of string tied round it … What he did was to hold the reel by the

> string and very skillfully throw it over the edge of his curtained cot, so that it disappeared into it, at the same time uttering his expressive 'o-o-o-o'. (1920: 15)

Freud agreed with the boy's mother that the child's utterance meant '*fort*' ('gone'). Freud continued his description: 'He then pulled the reel out of the cot again by the string and hailed its reappearance with a joyful "*da*" ["there"]. This, then, was the complete game – disappearance and return' (1920: 15). According to Freud, the child compensated himself for the instinctual renunciation he had made in allowing his mother to go away without protesting, 'by himself staging the disappearance and return of the objects within his reach ... The child cannot possibly have felt his mother's departure as something agreeable or even indifferent' (1920:15). Turning his experience into a game: 'At the outset he was in a *passive* situation – he was overpowered by the experience; but by repeating it, unpleasurable though it was, as a game, he took on an *active* part' (1920: 16). Freud's assessment of the goal or function of repetitive play was as follows:

> It is clear that in their play children repeat everything that has made a great impression on them in real life, and that in doing so they abreact the strength of the impression and ... make themselves master of the situation ... As the child passes over from the passivity of the experience to the activity of the game, he hands on the disagreeable experience to one of his playmates and in this way revenges himself on a substitute. (1920: 16–17)

Disappearance–return, here, is an example at an individual level of play, of inverted likeness expressing diametric structured behaviour and experience.

The diphasic pattern of reactive prohibition and substitutive satisfaction, as well as the mirror image inversion between passive and active roles, are features shared between medieval carnivals and festivals, on the one hand, and Freudian accounts of obsessional neurosis, on the other. Freud summarises a general feature of obsessional neurosis in terms that are tantamount to diametric mirror image inverted symmetry:

> The symptoms belonging to this [obsessional] neurosis fall, in general, into two groups, each having an opposite trend. They are either prohibitions, precautions and expiations – that is, negative in character – or they are, on the contrary, substitutive satisfactions which often appear in symbolic disguise. (1926: 112)

This builds on his observations in *Wolf Man*, of the interplay of two diametrically opposing states, 'sadistic aggressiveness towards the father and a tender passive attitude to him' that 'form a pair of opposites' (Freud 1926: 106).

Thus, an initial conclusion, building on this, would suggest that there is some tension between a Freudian potential characterisation of features of carnival and festival as diametric inverted symmetry of obsessional neurosis and Taylor's portrayal of the loss of carnival and festival's anti-structure role as a key contribution to the homogenisation of a secular time. The tension would not come from Freud's end, as he would presumably envisage development of a secular time as a movement from obsessional neurosis of religious rituals, but rather from Taylor's end, of search for a positive phenomenology of time to challenge the homogenous time of secularisation. Yet, it is not the diametric feature of inversion per se that leads to neurosis, for Freud, but rather its excessive repetition; diametric inversion is more a feature of ego identity formation.[8] Repetition and inversion are key features of play generally (Lancy 1980), so that in obsessional neurosis, these elements may be distinguished simply by the difference in degree of repetition and frequency of inversions.

In this light, Taylor's claim for loss of inversion in carnival, as key to development of a secular, homogenous time, can be interpreted as a view that diametric structures of mirror image symmetry, of inversion, are key dimensions to a non-secular and somehow transcendent time (and space). Yet this is a very big claim Taylor is making. There is supposedly something in this feature of inversion in carnival play and ritual that is lost in a secular society and in one reliant on a lived condition of homogenous time. This makes its entrance in Taylor's text as a quasi-epiphanic disclosure of meaning and further interrogation is required of what this, almost primordial, dimension could be.

In what sense could a dimension of transcendence, as a condition for lived experience, be located or associated with carnival inversion? Drawing out an implication of Taylor's claim, there is potentially some dimension here, which would go beyond simple cultural relativism; the game of carnival inversion is not to be a mere language game of Wittgenstein. The claim for carnival eschews a relativism and as it is at the level of the unthought of a culture, as a background horizon of assumption, carnival inversion is a prelinguistic mode of relation, loss of which leads to experience of a secular time.

Whereas Heidegger refers to a structure of being, as a background mode of relation, this *structural* dimension is somewhat underplayed by Taylor, in his search for hidden conditions, unless time could be expressed as being non-homogenous in some structural way. Derrida notes that Lévi-Strauss gave much attention in anthropology to play and games, with references 'notably to roulette', which are 'very frequent' (1978: 290). The danger with the language-games metaphor of Wittgenstein is that it makes a roulette of truths, random, relativistic and infinitely malleable, what Heidegger would term 'empty logical possibility' 1927/1962: 183). Taylor's archive on carnival inversion, as a potentially prelinguistic temporal mode of relation, views carnival not as an *ad hoc* roulette but as supposedly an expression of some pivotal underlying pattern, on the road to a lived condition of transcendence, or at least a life principle drawing on the Dionysian and the potential for a selfovercoming in the later Nietzsche.

Taylor's extrapolation of a pivotal role for loss of carnival, as loss of anti-structure and as a key condition for emergence of homogenous, secular time, relies on Turner's work on anti-structure for support. Moreover, building on Benedict Anderson's work on simultaneity in culture, Taylor comments:

> This very clear, unambiguous concept of simultaneity belongs to an understanding of time as exclusively secular. As long as secular time is interwoven with various kinds of higher time, there is no guarantee that all events can be placed in unambiguous relations of simultaneity and succession. The high feast is in one way contemporaneous with my life and that of my fellow pilgrims, but in another way it is close to eternity, or the time of origins, or the earth it prefigures. (2007: 209)

This is an interesting historical narrative on the origins of the development of homogenous time and secularism. Yet, interrogating a spatial discourse of relation in Taylor is not so much with respect to a past-based focus on origins of the construction of homogenous space, neither its relation to secularism directly, however revealing these accounts could be. While Taylor accentuates the temporal features of the carnival and festival period, an examination of this ritual of inversion, as a diametric mode of relation, introduces a spatial focus, as well, on carnival and this period as anti-structure.

Conditions or frames for experience in sociohistorical context are examined by Taylor in relation to time, through the vehicle of his conception of what he terms 'the social imaginary' (2007: 171), namely, 'the way ordinary people "imagine" their social surroundings, and this is often not expressed in theoretical terms, it is carried in images, stories, legends etc.' (2007: 171–172). As a background taken for granted 'common understanding which makes possible common practices and a widely shared sense of legitimacy' (2007: 172), Taylor's thought in relation to time in the 'social imaginary' accommodates a foreground–background kind of conceptualisation in examining these changing temporal frames in relation to experience of religious belief and secularism.

A further point made by Taylor, regarding the function of the inversion in carnival rituals, invites the implication that the inversion of carnival was not simply diametric space *simpliciter*:

> In rituals of reversal … we have not only the airing of opposed principles, which are allowed to emerge and engage in mock battle. The aim is frequently also to bring them to some kind of synergy; to make the structure less self-enclosed, and at the same time to allow it draw on the energy of anti-structure in order to renew itself. (2007: 53)

This suggested feature of a reciprocal complementarity of sorts between diametric opposites, for at least some inversions of role in some carnivals, would move the diametric inversion towards a Gestalt figure–ground relation, Wittgenstein's duck–rabbit.

It would seem that a backdrop for Taylor's assertions on 'the power of anti-structure' (2007: 50), that 'all structure needs anti-structure' (2007: 47) is in part Nietzsche's espousal of the antithetical force of Dionysus to Apollonian certainty in BT. As argued in Chapter 5, as mutually self-defining contrasts that do not overlap the same space but rather interact to a limited degree with one another, Nietzsche's Apollonian and Dionysian counterpoles give implicit expression to a predominant spatial structure of figure–ground interaction.

Nietzsche's 'ecstasy of the Dionysian state' (BT: 46) is a not so remote ancestor of Laing's (1967) excoriating attack on societal normality, where via Mallarmé, he referred to that estranged integration called normality as the abdication of ecstasy, a desiccated version of a presumably Apollonian state of normality that denies death by avoiding life, conning children out of play. In similar vein, loss of carnival and festival inversions is a putative conning of society out of play, as a Dionysian counterpole, as a condition for homogenous, secular time.

Nietzsche, the self-styled antimoralist, the antiChrist of *Ecce Homo*, the expounder of the antinomy between the Apollonian and Dionysian from *The Birth of Tragedy* onwards, is the diametrician *in extremis*. He accepts in *Ecce Homo* that inversion is almost his métier. While Apollo and Dionysus are conceived of as being complementary, as in 'the one-sided Apollonian "will"' (BT: 58) coexisting within a 'fraternal bond' (BT: 126), as though in a reciprocal figure–ground relation, other diametric relations rely on a conception of being 'anti'. Taylor offers a view of Nietzsche's famous polarities that implies they are in diametric figure–ground relation of mutual complementarity: 'This morality was the enemy of the controlled unleashing of the Will to Power, where the Apollonian order would be at the service of Dionysian force' (2007: 599).

Vertical interplay between concentric and diametric space as eternal recurrence includes a horizontal movement towards flattened homogenous space as monism for experience of time

Taylor invokes the Dionysian through medieval carnival to reinvigorate a flattened homogenous time in lived experience rather than a flattened space. Seeking to vivify experience, this is thereby an appeal to a life principle. Taylor locates the source of such a life principle in inversion, in the limited form of diametric mirror image symmetry of carnival.

Taylor's archive on rituals of carnival can be seen as a homogenous, secular time emerging through a double loss, from figure–ground diametric relation, via diametric relation *simpliciter*, to a flat monism: 'It was the eclipse of this sense of necessary complementarity, of the need for anti-structure, which preceded and helped to bring about the secularization of public space' (2007: 50). The spatial movement is from monism to diametric relation *simpliciter* to figure–ground diametric relation, with concentric spatial modes of assumed connection to possibly come on the horizon.

Reversing Taylor's historically focused direction of movement from diametric inversion to monism as loss of conditions for experience supporting religious belief, a fundamental spatial directional focus places the direction of movement from monism towards diametric spatial inversion and after to concentric relation with each prior dimension mediating the one that follows. Appositely for Taylor's concerns, this spatial directionality implicates a *temporal* direction of movement. Such temporality of fundamental spatial movements is not identical to linear time, all the while that it commingles with its material events and patterns within linear history.

These temporal directions in interplay gives further flesh to Nietzsche's eternal recurrence as dynamic interplay between concentric and diametric spatial movements; these spaces interact with a mediating mode of figure–ground spatial relations. In addition to the vertical movements of eternal recurrence as concentric and diametric spatial directions, a horizontal movement towards monism takes place. This is the horizontal movement observed by Taylor as the flattened monism for time, if not space; Taylor perceives, at least indirectly, the flattening of diametric space into monism, although not the *écrasement* of concentric space, whether into diametric space or a further shift into a spatial monism. A monism of homogenous space loses the primordial experiential capacity for symmetry, whether the symmetry as unity of concentric space or the inverted mirror image symmetry of diametric space.

Taylor's words that: 'It is out of lived experience that we either find the way to break out of the Iron Cage, or to transfigure the world of ennui, or to reconnect the lost time' (2007: 720) can be adapted to this distinctive spatial focus. A key immersion in lived experience of the moment can help move out of the iron cage of diametric spatially structured experience towards a concentric space that is less a lost space from the past as a potential space for engagement in the moment.

A potential has been outlined for a temporal movement between monism, diametric space *simpliciter*, figure–ground diametric relation towards a concentric spatial relation underlying lived conditions for experience relevant to change to homogenous flattened space underpinning experience of time. This provides potential increments of expansion as parts of horizons of futurity and not only history. Significantly, movement can potentially be in both spatial directions along this axis. This movement can be viewed as two kinds of 'death' of diametric space, one in the direction of monism of homogenous space, the other in the direction of concentric spatial relation.

Notes

1 Schopenhauer is likewise also locked within the diametric opposition of the ideal versus real: '[W]e found in the first book that the correct starting-point for philosophy is essentially and necessarily the subjective, i.e., the idealistic, just as the opposite starting-point, proceeding from the objective, leads to materialism' (WWR II: 486). Even while he recognises 'the delusion that could separate' (WWR II: 486) the will in itself from phenomenal world of appearances, 'seeing through the *principium individuationis*' (WWR II: 606), he does not offer a relation beyond either monistic fusion as unity or diametric opposition.

2 Muneto suggests that: 'The idea [of eternal recurrence] is not to be communicated by way of a ladder of concepts or logic, nor is it presented as something complete in itself. It wants to be perceived intuitively and guessed both in the process as it gradually arises and also at the moment when it "flashes"' (1991: 234). For Parkes, Nietzsche's psychology is 'above all imagistic, a discipline practised in images rather than in concepts', especially Zarathustra (1994: 7), where eternal recurrence is particularly developed.

3 As described in Downes: '[T]he flattened line is derivative from the circle. A line requires additional resources to emerge to be a circle. A circle contains the potential of a line within itself, as a loss of its circularity, whereas a line does not contain the potential of a circle within itself, without addition. In this spatial logic, a circle is more fundamental or primordial than the line' (2012: 337).

4 Krell's footnote (1991: 41, Vol. II) associates this moment with Heidegger's ecstatic temporality in *Being and Time*. See also Downes (2012) for an interpretation of Heidegger's ecstatic temporality in *Being and Time* in terms of concentric and diametric spaces, including linear time as inauthentic temporality as a diametric spatial projection.

5 See Downes (2012) for the development of these different levels in terms of Heidegger's conception of temporality as the horizon for the question of being.

6 See, for example, Lévi-Strauss, *Structural Anthropology, Vol. 1*, 151.

7 See Downes (2012) for an account of this debate.

8 See Downes, P., 'Cross-Cultural Structures of Concentric and Diametric Dualism in Lévi-Strauss's Structural Anthropology: Structures of Relation Underlying the Self and Ego Relation?', *Journal of Analytical Psychology*, 2003, *48*: 47–81.

References

Bertram, E., *Nietzsche. Attempt at a Mythology*. Trans. R. E. Norton. Urbana/Chicago, IL: University of Illinois Press, 1919/2009.

Clark, M. and Dudrick, D., *The Soul of Nietzsche's 'Beyond Good and Evil'*. Cambridge: Cambridge University Press, 2012.

Derrida, J., *Of Grammatology*. London/Baltimore: Johns Hopkins University Press, 1974.

Derrida, J., *Writing and Difference*. Trans. A. Bass. London: Routledge & Kegan Paul, 1978/1981.

Derrida, J., *The Post Card: From Socrates to Freud and Beyond*. Trans. A. Bass. Chicago, IL: University of Chicago Press, 1987.

Downes, P., 'Schema Structure-Content Relativity: Part II, From Image Schemata to Background Spatial Schemata of Diametric and Concentric Relation;, *Cybernetics and Human Knowing*, 2010,17: 25–43.

Downes, P., *The Primordial Dance: Diametric and Concentric Spaces in the Unconscious World*. Oxford/Bern: Peter Lang, 2012.

Freud, S., *Beyond the Pleasure Principle*. SE 18. London: Hogarth Press, 1920.
Freud, S., *Inhibitions, Symptoms and Anxiety*. SE20. London: Hogarth Press, 1926.
Heidegger, M., *Being and Time*. Trans. J. MacQuarrie and E. Robinson. Oxford: Basil Blackwell, 1927/1962.
Heidegger, M., *Nietzsche*, Vols and IV. D. F. Krell (ed.), trans. J. Stambaugh, D. F. Krell and F. A. Capuzzi. New York: HarperCollins, 1987.
Heidegger, M., *Nietzsche*, Vols I and II. D. F. Krell (ed.), trans. D. F. Krell. New York: HarperCollins, 1991.
Hofstadter, D.R., *Godel, Escher, Bach: An Eternal Golden Braid*. New York: Basic Books, 1979.
James, W., *The Principles of Psychology*. New York: Holt, 1890.
Janaway, C., 'Nietzsche's Psychology as a Refinement of Plato's', *Journal of Nietzsche Studies*, 2014, 45: 12–21.
Kaufmann, W., *Nietzsche: Philosopher, Psychologist, Antichrist,* 4th ed. Princeton, NJ: Princeton University Press, 1975.
Kerenyi, C., *Dionysus: Archetypal Image of Indestructible Life*. Princeton, NJ: Princeton University Press, 1976.
Krell, D. F.. 'Introduction to Martin Heidegger, *Nietzsche*' (Vols I and II). D. F.Krell (ed.), trans. D. F. Krell. New York: HarperCollins, 1991.
Laing, R. D., *The Politics of Experience*. London: Penguin, 1967.
Lancy, D. F., 'Play in Species Adaptation', *Annual Review of Anthropology*, 1980, 9: 471–495.
Lévi-Strauss, C., *The Savage Mind*. Rrans. G. Weidenfeld, Nicolson Ltd. Chicago, IL: Chicago University Press, 1962/1966.
Lévi-Strauss, C., *Structural Anthropology*, Vol. 1. Trans. C. Jacobsen and B. Grundfest Schoepf. London: Penguin, 1963.
Lévi-Strauss, C., *The Raw and the Cooked: Introduction to a Science of Mythology* I. London: Jonathan Cape, 1970.
Lévi-Strauss, C., *Structural Anthropology*, Vol. 2. Trans. M. Layton. London: Penguin Books, 1973/1977.
Muneto, S., 'The Eloquent Silence of Zarathustra by Sonoda Muneto' (trans. S. Aihara and G. Parkes), in G. Parkes (ed.), *Nietzsche and Asian Thought*. Chicago, IL: University of Chicago Press, 1991.
Parkes, G., *Composing the Soul: Reaches of Nietzsche's Psychology*. Chicago, IL: University of Chicago Press, 1994.
Taylor, C., *A Secular Age*. Cambridge, MA: Harvard University Press, 2007.
Turner, V., *The Ritual Process: Structure and Anti-Structure*. Ithaca, NY: Cornell University Press, 1969.
Turner, V., *The Ritual Process: Structure and Anti-Structure Dramas, Fields and Metaphors*. Ithaca, NY: Cornell University Press, 1978.

Chapter 9

Space prior to metaphor

Spatial understandings and assumptions pervade much of Ricoeur's discussion of metaphor in terms of proximity and distance, tension, substitution, interaction, displacement, change of location, assimilation, image, the 'open' structure of words, transparency and opaqueness. Again and again, space emerges and inserts itself into Ricoer's concerns. Yet this is usually where space is discussed within metaphor, and as a metaphor itself, rather than as a precondition or prior system of relations to language interacting with language.

At the core of Ricoeur's interrogation in *La Métaphore Vive*, his search is for a living metaphor, a metaphor that lives, an animating principle underpinning and arguably prior to metaphor. It is a life principle in MV that is in some way so obvious and foregrounded, it becomes too close to be fully seen, a life principle that is not aided for viewing by the distorting lens of translation of *La Métaphore Vive* from life, from metaphor as living, to the more inert terminology of rule, *The Rule of Metaphor*. This translational slippage from life to rule moves the angle of preoccupation with and interpretation of this work away from life and the primordial, and towards interrogation of speech acts and rules in the analytic philosophy of Austin, Searle and colleagues. Thus, a life principle in Ricoeur becomes hidden in full view, so to speak.

Ricoeur seeks to expand the ambit of relevance for metaphor from the word to the sentence to discourse, through a broadening of conceptions of reference. He seeks to suspend primary reference of truth as correspondence to an external world in science and to invoke a split reference to encompass another referential domain for metaphor in discourse, a 'world' or state of affairs of poetic reference. This reconstruction of referential relevance for metaphor in discourse requires a shift beyond the familiar terrain of the dichotomies between sense and reference, connotation and denotation. Yet this broadening of the scope of metaphor almost goes a step further to embrace an expansion of the role of space beyond simply existing within metaphor. Ricoeur treats the spatialisation of language that is itself a language of space as a 'brilliant maxim' (MV: 147) of Genette.

In Study 6 of MV, Ricoeur also arrives at the threshold of a spatial questioning when invoking Bachelard to raise the question of a verbal mode that is vassal to the nonverbal (MV: 214). As well as relying on spatially imbued concepts throughout, Ricoeur arrives at several thresholds of space, but stops short at delving further into these spaces. In MV, Ricoeur begins to trace the contours of a path regarding space as itself a discourse and system interacting with language but he does not walk through this pathway. This chapter seeks to open up the contours of this spatial pathway that is tantamount to being a promissory note in MV. Diametric and concentric spaces are not argued to be metaphors but rather prior structures of relation to metaphor, actively framing metaphor.

In developing the concept of metaphorical truth in Study 7 of MV, Ricoeur seeks a 'primary focus' on 'the "is" of equivalence' (MV: 248). Whereas Ricoer's explicit consideration of Heidegger in MV tends to focus on some of his later works on metaphor, such as *Der Satz vom Grund* and *Unterwegs zur Sprache*, the current spatial interrogation seeks structures of being, purportedly more primordial than metaphor. It is notable that Ricoeur does invoke a conception linking primordiality with space in relation to speculative discourse, which he describes as 'the discourse that establishes the primary notions, the principles that articulate primordially the space of the concept' (MV: 300). The further step being made here in terms of concentric and diametric spaces is to uncover this space as prior to language, as an autonomous system of meaning and relations, as a precondition for language to be.

Arguably resonant with Ricoeur's declared 'ontological aim' of carrying 'the metaphorical utterance back to the copula, understood in the sense of being-as' (MV: 257), the proposed prior space exists not simply within metaphor as a metaphor but as a silent discourse framing conditions for metaphor to be. Arguments for the relevance of concentric and diametric spaces to Derrida's quest for a new psychoanalytic graphology, embracing Freudian and Jungian thought, as well as to frames for moral reasoning have been emphasised elsewhere (Downes 2003, 2012, 2013). Moreover, it is argued elsewhere that concentric and diametric spaces are not reducible to image schemata or conceptual metaphors but rather that these are displaced forms of these prior spaces (Downes 2010, 2012).

The current argument will focus on establishing the relevance of this proposed prior, prelinguistic spatial discourse between diametric and concentric structures to Ricoeur's framework of metaphor and interrogation of the copula influenced centrally by Heidegger. In doing so, it will seek to foreground the relevance of this spatial interplay to aspects of Ricoeur's thought, especially in MV, thereby amplifying issues touched on regarding Ricoeur's thought, although resting largely implicit there.

A number of entailments of the relative differences between concentric and diametric spaces have been identified in previous chapters: contrasts between i) assumed separation (diametric space) and assumed connection (concentric space), ii) symmetry as mirror image inversion (diametric space) and symmetry as unity (concentric space) and iii) relative closure from background (diametric space) compared with relative openness to background (concentric space). Only the last two entailments were recognised by Lévi-Strauss. In this chapter, most focus, although not all, will be on i). In Bachelard's words, pertinent to diametric space, 'simple geometrical opposition becomes tinged with aggressivity' (1964: 212).

The proposed concentric and diametric spatial contrasts between assumed connection and separation help overcome what Ricoeur describes as the 'ruinous distinction' (MV: 234) between cognition and emotion. D'Aquili (1975) notes the Cartesian commitments of Lévi-Strauss to uncovering mental structures; it may have been these very commitments to rigid Cartesian dichotomies that led to Lévi-Strauss' blind spot for this key entailment that concentric relation challenges such dichotomies and is more connective than diametric relation.

A concentric model of inwardness allows for an inner realm that is not reducible to the outer but which is in a relation of assumed connection with it. It also allows for a conception of an inner realm of experience that is not necessarily a detached abstraction from the outer in Cartesian fashion. When discussing resemblance and 'the kind of semantic "proximity" established between the terms despite their "distance" apart', Ricoeur invokes the 'metaphor of "far" and "near"' and seeks a preconceptual generic relatedness 'to suppress distance [*dés-éloigner*].'(MV: 194). This is highly resonant with an interplay between concentric assumed connection and diametric assumed separation. It is important to emphasise that concentric relation of assumed connection as nearness or proximity is not the same as identity as equivalence; it is not a monistic relation. A concentric relation allows for distinction and difference that does not have to lead to opposition. Difference is maintained but through a conjoined relation of assumed connection between concentric poles. It is this assumed connection that echoes Ricoeur's concern with belongingness. Significantly, Ricoeur invokes a relational conception of 'primordial belonging' (MV: 306) as a background understanding for discourse and metaphorical truth.

Concentric space offers a conceptualisation of Ricoeur's sought for as-structure of belonging for metaphor, which expresses a relation of both identity and difference through a framing mode of assumed connection. Concentric spatial relation as a mode of identity-cum-difference offers a response to Ricoeur's question of how to reconcile similarity and sameness (MV: 192), building on Aristotle's characterisation in poetics of a good metaphor as an intuitive perception of similarity in dissimilars.

With strong echoes of Heidegger, Ricoeur's interrogation of metaphor as a problem of identity and difference in relation to being and to the question of being as including an 'is not' within a predicative assertion of 'is' leads to Ricoeur's spatial acknowledgment of a 'topology of being' for Heidegger that again chimes with Ricoeur's concerns with 'nearness of the "near"' in 'the play of resemblance' (MV: 309) in metaphor. Ricoeur explores the as-structure of being-as, and belonging-as to examine a space for play around identity that is not necessarily equivalence.

Elsewhere in his work, a spatial insight of Ricoeur further opens the door to addressing this blind spot in the spatial structural understandings of Lévi-Strauss concerning assumed connection and separation in his cross-cultural observations of diametric and concentric structures. Ricoeur (HHS) refers to an implicitly spatial preunderstanding of 'distanciation' as establishing the relation between subject and object. He treats distanciation as the reflective, critical or suspicious moment within consciousness; such a spatial concern with distanciation is tantamount to an implicit spatial logic as the seed of a spatial discourse not yet unfolded. While the assumed separation of diametric relation is not to be equated with Ricoeur's concept of distanciation, nevertheless, both perspectives on the subject–object relation recognise a fundamental distance or separation – a spatial conception – as the basis for the subject–object dualism.

Ricoeur explicitly appeals to Heidegger's being-in-the-world as the basis for a contrast to distanciation – a contrast which Ricoeur terms 'belonging' (MV: 110/51). Ricoeur treats belonging as an immediate or unreflective relation 'correcting' distanciation and a concretizing of the universality of distanciation. Diametric spatial relation is thus resonant with Ricoeur's distanciation underlying the subject–object relation as diametric spatial relation involves an entailment of assumed separation. In contrast, the belonging of concentric relation involves an entailment of assumed connection between its poles. While these relative differences between concentric and diametric spaces may be observed empirically, these inferences are being envisaged as *a priori* entailments. They are not being derived from empirical examples; the examples are simply illustrative. The inferences are of relative priority, a necessity of relative priority.

It is recognized that transcendental, *a priori* arguments are, as Körner (1967) exposes, always vulnerable with regard to the strong Kantian claim for their necessity. A claim for necessity cannot exclude myriad other possible circumstances. It is not being argued that the relative differences between concentric and diametric structures meet a strong Kantian claim for absolute necessity. Rather, it is a specific contextual necessity of relative priority. They are directional contrasts rather than static positional truth claims treating each space in isolation from the other. As relative differences, a vital directional dimension to assumptions of connection and separation is embraced. They are only positional structures relative to each other, rather than in an absolute essentialist spatial sense. They are also relativistic, directional projections. In other words, their operationalisations would be meaningless without the counterpole; it is a relation that is being operationalised, a directional relation (whether towards an assumed connection or separation).

The issue is not so much one of uncovering a 'substance' but rather a dynamic relationship. As projections, these spaces are dynamic structures and active processes, as well as describing functions of relation. These relative differences are not, to adapt Ricoeur's words in a different context, a 'system of associated commonplaces' (MV: 169); they are not argued to be simply empirical cultural constructions[1] but are inferences based on the structural contrasts between these spaces. These are not private images in the sense that Ricoeur refers to images (MV: 208, 2011) but rather publicly justifiable inferences from these spatial-structural contrasts.[2]

It is important to emphasise that this framework of a system of relations between concentric and diametric spatial discourse is to be distinguished from not only other structuralist commitments generally in Lévi-Strauss' work – but also from being related to what Ricoeur terms the 'binarist zeal' (MV: 174) of Jakobson's structuralism. The range and level of inferences between concentric and diametric spaces offer a multidimensional framework far from simple binarism, while also directly challenging the binarism of diametric spaces.

This concern with a spatial phenomenology of relation through concentric and diametric spaces has antecedents already in French phenomenology (and not only French structuralism via Lévi-Strauss), such as Bachelard's recognition that: 'Philosophers, when confronted with outside and inside, think in terms of being and non-being. Thus profound metaphysics is rooted in an implicit geometry which – whether we will or no – confers spatiality upon thought' (1964: 212). Ricoeur explicitly notes Bachelard's phenomenological position where the image dominates over language (MV: 214). However, this phenomenology *through* space in concentric and diametric spatial relations is to be distinguished from Bachelard's evocative phenomenology of space and of objects in space.

Bachelard's lens of concentration is mainly on physical perceptual spaces in a 'phenomenology of images' (1964: 112) whereas a phenomenology *through* space is a spatial–relational concern with unconscious structures projected into experience. Concentric and diametric spaces are argued to pertain also to ontological dimensions. In contrast, with implicit reference to Heidegger's existential phenomenology, Bachelard acknowledges that: 'Such formulas as being-in-the-world [...] are too majestic for me and I do not succeed in experiencing them [...] I feel more at home in miniature worlds' (1964: 161). It is with this wider world pertaining to structures of being that a spatial-phenomenological lens of concentric and diametric spaces can come to the fore.

Other key entailments of the multidimensional contrasts between diametric and concentric primordial spaces: inverted symmetry/symmetry as unity, closure/openness

Ricoeur's concerns touch briefly on issues of symmetry in metaphor (MV: 198) including symmetry by inversion (MV: 234), whereas Lévi-Strauss explicitly relates concrete spatial diametric structures to mirror image symmetrical inversions between both diametric poles. While Lévi-Strauss related diametric structured, mirror image symmetry to myths and sought 'unconscious' (1963: 53) structures, he did not integrate this with a detailed examination of this structure's relevance to wider emotions, beyond a recognition of affect underlying attributions such as good and bad. Concentric spatial structures of relation are not symmetry as inversion. Rather they offer a different entailment of symmetry as unity, where the line or axis of symmetry brings the same pole rather than a mirror image pole in diametric structures.

Again Ricoeur raises what are tantamount to spatial concerns regarding metaphor in terms of an 'open structure' (MV: 170) to words, as well as considerations of 'closure' (MV: 126). These can gain further flesh through consideration of a third entailment of the relative differences between concentric and diametric spaces – open foreground–background interaction versus relatively closed noninteraction. Diametric structures' relation to their own poles is one of a mirror image division, which then maintains a cleavage from the background that becomes closed off. Moreover, diametric and concentric structures are dynamic processes as much as structures. Thus, a diametric structure tends to impose a diametric process in its interaction with the background, whereas a concentric structure initiates a concentric relation with the background.

In this sense of involvement with the background, concentric relation is not a self-contained structure. There is a closer proximity between background and foreground within concentric relative to diametric space. In comparison, diametric space is a much more closed structure – closed off from the background. There is greater closure in a diametric spatial structure relative to a dis-closure process of relative opening in concentric spatial relation.

A variant of the entailment of relative closure for diametric structures is that they bring decreased permeability and transparency relative to the increased permeability and transparency of concentric structures. Key features of metaphor, highlighted by Ricoeur, such as tension, substitution and interaction, are all aspects of the tension between concentric and diametric spaces. Movement between these spaces allows not only for interaction between them but also of replacement of one space by another, akin to a mode of substitution. The relative openness and permeability of concentric structural relations offer a background for Ricoeur's consideration of transparency for metaphor, which he contrasts with opacity (MV: 145). This offers a further resonance with the more closed structures of diametric space. Interplay between concentric and diametric spaces offers a more differentiated understanding of the actively engaged role of space in experience than a flat, one-size-fits-all characterisation of space as the void of nothingness.

Ricoeur's objections to Heidegger's critique of the metaphysical within the metaphorical and to Jakobson's selection-combination binarism: issues for the proposed spatial discourse of concentric and diametric structures of relation

A notable tension exists between Ricoeur and Heidegger on the issue of Heidegger's well-known contention that the metaphorical only exists within the metaphysical, being locked within a sensory/nonsensory opposition of Western metaphysical traditions of thought.[3] One limb of Ricoeur's objection is based on a proportionality principle, when recognising that: 'The distinction between proper and figurative meaning applied to individual words is an obsolete semantic notion that does not have to be tacked onto metaphysics to be taken to pieces' (MV: 282). Ricoeur additionally contests the equivalence of the two transfers, the metaphysical transfer from the sensible to the nonsensible, the metaphorical transfer from the literal to the figurative. Furnishing his argument with concrete examples,[4] Ricoeur seeks a wider notion of metaphor than one reduced simply to visible/invisible oppositions.

Ricoeur's challenge here is at a content level of specific exceptions in metaphor to the sensory–nonsensory, or at least visible–invisible binary opposition; a further step is to overcome this oppositional structure itself, in other words, to move from a diametric spatial relation of mirror image inverted symmetry between the sensory and nonsensory. Interpreted as a spatial shift away from diametric structures of relation, the question arises as to the existence of a concentric spatial relation to engage the sensory and to refashion the traditional metaphysical opposition between the sensory and nonsensory. This invites further scrutiny of the role of space underpinning the sensory realm, to transform understandings of the sensory.[5] Space relates fundamentally to the presensory, as a precondition for the sensory.

Space is not simply as an object for the sensory, to be seen, heard as silence, touched, smelled and tasted. Moreover, the contours of space are not simply as a contrastive point of reference for experience of the sensory, where James (1890) highlights the sound of thunder as requiring a background of silence; space can be but is not solely in a diametric mirror image opposition to sound or other senses, as a passive background. More significantly, space can also be understood actively as an inner concentric dimension, within which senses are embedded, as an inner connective precondition, for example, for sound. Without the medium of space, sound cannot be heard; without space to move through, the resistance of touch cannot be experienced.

This is not to deny the key role of the sensory in projecting experiences of sight, sound, touch, taste and smell into language for the metaphorical (see, e.g. Derrida 1985, 2005 on the haptic and the ear of the other); it is additionally to interrogate projection of a prior realm of diametric and concentric spaces underpinning experience and language. This is not merely a quest for an animating space to modify abstraction in the nonsensory; it is fundamentally an interrogation of the surreptitious immanence of primordial space as concentric relations. In his critique of Heidegger regarding the metaphysical in the metaphorical, a key search of Ricoeur is for a mode of metaphor *to escape the diametric sensory–nonsensory opposition, or at least visible–invisible opposition of metaphysics.*

Concern for current purposes is with a spatial mode of experience *prior to the sensory*, projected into language and thought, that does not seek to escape from the meta, i.e., beyond, of the metaphysical and meta*phorical*; it is for a spatial mode of experience that shifts the diametric mirror image split spatial structure from being a supporting precondition underpinning the meta (in both the metaphysical and metaphorical), into a different embedded spatial mode of concentric relation. Ricoeur offers a range of fundamental metaphors, such as the heliotrope, home, return, all of which are amenable to understanding in concentric spatial modes – the sun as a concentric radial structure, dwelling alongside as the concentric home of assumed connection, return as projection of a common spatial structural movement of both concentric and diametric space propagating their respective modes of relation.

Elsewhere it has been argued that such a concentric spatial mode of experience, prior to the sensory, can be located in the breath, as part of a shift from a mind–body (nonsensory–sensory) opposition to a breath–body opposition (Downes 2012).[6] In other words, experience of concentric and diametric spaces as assumed connection and separation, as relative openness and closure, are meaningful for meditative experience of the breath immersed in the body, as a more fundamental primordial mode of experience, prior to the sensory.

Concentric space offers a presensuous emptiness, a presensuous intuition of an active emptiness for the breath flow, as distinct from a Cartesian emptiness as nonentity. This presensuous mode of experience is not nonsensuous; concentric spatial relations can be projected also into and through the senses. This proposed spatial protolanguage of silence brings an emptying of language as a path to meaning prior to language, peopled by spaces too bright to see, to adapt Shelley in *Prometheus Unbound.*

The diametric space of mirror image inversion underpins Western metaphysics, through its sensory–nonsensory opposition framing the metaphysical and founding abstraction; the unseating of this diametric space through concentric space is at issue. Ricoeur contests the equivalence of the two transfers, the metaphysical transfer from the sensible to the nonsensible, the metaphorical transfer from the literal to the figurative; that these transfers reveal a common precondition of diametric space, as mirror image inverted symmetry, is not to assert the equivalence of these transfers but it is to highlight the structural commonality of a potentially malleable governing spatial precondition. Ricoeur's interrogation of analogy as onto-theology, where he seeks for analogy to retain 'its own conceptual structure' (MV: 270) through entering the problematic of being, offers another example of metaphysics as diametric spatial inverted symmetry. With regard to analogy in relation to metaphor, again a diametric mirror image relation of inversion emerges in Ricoeur's account of St Thomas Aquinas on this issue:

> The question of metaphor is confronted head on in the *Summa Theologiae* (1 a, qu 13, art. 6) under the question: 'Whether names predicated of God are predicated primarily of creatures?' The answer distinguishes two orders of priority: a priority according to the thing itself, which begins with what is first in itself, that is, God; and a priority according to signification, which begins with what is best known to us, that is, creatures. The first type of priority governs analogy properly speaking and the second, metaphor. (MV: 278)

Ricoeur continues:

> This intersection of two kinds of transference, following the descending order of being and the ascending order of significations, explains the creation of composite modalities of discourse in which the meaning effects of proportional metaphor and transcendental analogy are added together [...] One rests on the predication of transcendental terms, the other on the predication of meanings that carry their material content with them. (MV: 279–280)

This scholastic concern with intersection of contrasting directions of transcendental analogy and metaphor as *proportionalitas*, i.e., a resemblance of relations between any terms whatever (as distinct from *proportio* here), again relies on the diametric mirror image inversion between ascent–descent, transcendental–material. This whole framing of the discussion of analogy operates against the backdrop of a structural presupposition of the metaphysical. A different spatial structural underpinning is needed than the metaphysical structure underpinning this analogy–metaphor relation, reliant on a diametric spatial reversal between ascent–descent, material–transcendent.[7]

This raises the question of an alternative background space to diametric relations, such as concentric space. This spatial background needs to supply a different spatial-structural underpinning, through which analogy can operate (whether as a unitary or heterogeneous structure), although the task of developing this spatial questioning for analogy is beyond the scope of this book. Ricoeur raises a further concern with a core feature of the structural linguistics of Jakobson that is also an apt question for current purposes. Resonant with Saussure, Jakobson (1971) treats any and all linguistic entities as involving two modes of arrangement, namely combination and selection.

Ricoeur suggests that :

> [T]he strength of Jakobson's schema is also its weakness. The strength of the bipolar scheme lies in its extreme generality and its extreme simplicity [...] a heavy price must be paid [...] when applied to the domain of rhetoric, the binarism of the schema needlessly restricts its field to two figures [...] The notion is too wide when one considers the heterogeneity of substitution and selection operations from one level to another [...] [with] no place for the phenomenon of interaction, specifically of metaphorical statements, in the orbit of the selection-substitution phenomenon. (MV: 178–179)

From a similar vantage point, it might be asked whether the proposed spatial discourse of concentric and diametric structures of relation is, at once, both too narrowly restrictive and too wide to encompass heterogeneity.

It has already been emphasised that the entailments of the relational contrasts between concentric and diametric spaces are multidimensional, so it is not simply a binary reduction. Moreover, although initially drawn from Lévi-Strauss' structuralist observations of a compensatory relation between these spaces, entailments of the relations between concentric and diametric spaces are not confined to the procrustean bed of structuralism, whether that of Lévi-Strauss or Jakobson. As claims for primordial spaces, this is a concern with a unity within experience;[8] it is not a universalist truth totality claim for all spaces, all experiences, all language, such as the totalising claim for language of Jakobson's bipolar categories.

As spaces in mutual dynamic interactive tension, concentric and diametric spaces are not merely static categories side-by-side with one another; neither are they static grounds for truth claims. In *Being and Time*, Heidegger raises the question of the dynamic background horizon between categories and *existentialia*. As William J. Richardson highlights, it is a question of being: 'It is only when we comprehend the horizon of transcendence as both the unifying dynamism of sheer presence and as non-being that we understand it properly' (1974: 148). This invites the question as to the background relation itself between concentric and diametric spaces. Envisaged as diametric categories side-by-side with one another, there would be an assumed separation of noninteraction between diametric and concentric spaces. However, if the relation itself between concentric and diametric spaces operates through a further concentric background horizon of assumed connection, this would allow for a more dynamic interplay between the spaces.[9] Such an interactive directional horizon between the proposed primordial spaces opens them from being static categories and from a premature positional grounding of these spaces, towards being directional horizons of possibility.

It is notable that the role envisaged by Ricoeur for his speculative discourse, is one where this is 'the horizon' (MV: 300) offering 'the gravitational pull' (MV: 64) on the referential concerns of metaphor. Ricoeur seeks an expansive spatial horizon as the gravitational pull to bring metaphor to life, with its 'dynamic, directional, vectoral character' (MV: 299) as a vivifying principle. The very image of gravitation here further invites spatial assumptions, with the recognition since Einstein, of gravitation as a curvature of space rather than a simple force *per se*.

Further resonance with Ricoeur here is his interrogation of a dialectical interplay between speculative discourse as the horizon and metaphorical discourse; the dynamic mutual interplay between concentric and diametric spaces, against the backdrop of a potentially dynamic, connective horizontal background of relation, gives further succour to Ricoeur's search for a greater dynamism than the static, all-embracing categories of Jakobson's overly reductive selection–combination opposition. In his search for an interactive dynamism beyond the schematic, Ricoeur goes so far as to refer to the 'containment of metaphorical discourse by speculative discourse' (MV: 302) thereby implying a concentric relation of containment and assumed connection between the two spheres. Yet Ricoeur also accepts that speculative discourse offers 'a beginning in itself and [...] the principle of its articulation within itself [...] that articulate[s] primordially the space of the concept' (MV: 300) in a further affinity with the spatial discourse of concentric and diametric structures of relation.

Rather than static binary categories, concentric and diametric spaces are argued elsewhere (Downes 2012) to be in dynamic interplay across a range of mutually interconnecting levels; these levels include Heidegger's basic ontological spaces, together with the background dynamic horizon for the question of being to connect these spaces interactively, as well as a further ontic level that encompasses referential concerns.[10] Put simply, at the ontic level of metaphor in language, a displacement of concentric and diametric spaces from the ontological level becomes a starting point for interrogation of these complex relations.

On the issue of the proposed spatial discourse encompassing heterogeneity, as argued elsewhere,[11] the work of Lakoff and Johnson has identified a range of conceptual metaphors and image schemata that offer structures as a key candidate, at the ontic level, for being displacements of the interplay between concentric and diametric spaces and their entailments of assumed connection–separation, symmetry–mirror image symmetry and openness–closure. The container schema is an illustrative but by no means sole example of spatial structures to encompass a heterogeneity of metaphors that is relevant also to a spatial discourse of concentric and diametric structures of relation. Lakoff and Johnson make explicit the 'built-in spatial "logics"' of the container schema, namely, that 'Given two containers, A and B, and an object X, if A is in B and X is in A, then X is in B' (1999: 31). They expand on the dimensions of this cross-modal image schema that is conceptual and yet can be physically instantiated:

> A container schema has the following structure: an inside, a boundary, and an outside [...] the parts make no sense without the whole. There is no inside without a boundary and an outside, no outside without a boundary and an inside, and no boundary without sides. (1999: 32)

Concentric spatial relation is a fundamental example of containment, where the inner pole is contained within the outer, unlike diametric space where neither pole contains the other. The spatial discourse of boundaries and containment underlying conceptual metaphor is a precursor to a wider, more fundamental spatial discourse of concentric and diametric spaces that can also encompass the heterogeneity of diverse conceptual metaphors.

Beyond metaphor to concentric and diametric space as a system of meaning prior to language as protolanguage

Metaphor emerges as part of a wider tension between primordial spaces. Ricoeur's question about 'what constitutes the metaphoricity of metaphor?' (MV: 193) can be met with a response that a prior spatial system of relations through diametric and concentric spaces are at least a necessary precondition for metaphor. Against the backdrop of this spatial discourse, the question can be reframed as to what constitutes the process of literalisation of meaning through the suppression of spatial movement and interplay.

A number of implications of this prior spatial system of relations emerge for language. Space is a precondition for language; language is not a precondition for space. Space is itself a system, a system of meaningful relations through the contrasts between diametric and concentric spaces. Space cannot be eliminated from language as a system of meaningful relations. The literal is an excess on the spatial. Rather than treating the space of metaphor as deviant or at least, deviation, it is the literal that is the excessive limiting condition. The literal is the line on the curve, the flattening of the space of the circle, the compression and concession of the space, where the diametric stasis of opposition is a process of tightening and tension to give meaning through difference.

In developing the concept of metaphorical truth in Study 7 of MV, Ricoeur builds on understanding of 'to be like–as' as a 'metaphorical modality of the copula itself'; Ricoeur emphasises the importance of preserving the 'is not' within the 'is' (MV: 249) in the copula in metaphorical statements. Concentric spatial relations of assumed connection allow for this distinction within identity to be preserved, although it is a more proximate relation than diametric spatial relations of firm difference and opposition, importing externality to difference. Concentric assumed connection and diametric assumed separation offer a framework for understanding, in Ricoeur's words the 'conflict between identity and difference' (MV: 198) in metaphor and beyond.

Ricoeur seeks to generalise 'a semantic phenomenon, assimilation to each other of two networks of signification by means of an unusual attribution' (MV: 198) in his account of resemblance underpinning metaphor. Again here 'assimilation' presupposes a spatial frame of understanding in relation to identity and difference, such as the silent glue of concentric space bringing the relation of assumed connection, while respecting difference between the two linguistic networks of signification in the metaphor. The background space of relation frames the assumption of connection between two initially diverse, disconnected networks of signification; they are moved from a diametric side-by-side assumption of basic separation towards one of concentric assumed connection in the metaphoric relation.

The structural interplay between concentric and diametric spaces operates as a background condition underpinning the tension between same and other, marking the relational copula. It is not a monism collapsing the identity of one part of a metaphorical 'to be like–as' statement into the other. With language as part of a wider tension between primordial spaces, space and language are part of a mutually embedded interconnected system of relations. Language needs space to breathe and be given life. Concentric and diametric spaces can go beyond a rational–affective dichotomy to reveal a discourse of implication that incorporates both reason and emotion.

Ricoeur's 'plea for the plurality of modes of discourse' (MV: 7) is, in effect, extended to this prelinguistic spatial discourse between concentric and diametric spaces. In developing the meaningfulness of a prelinguistic spatial discourse as a system of relations, at one level, it can be stated that this argument seeks to do to Lévi-Strauss, what Lévi-Strauss' structuralism does to Saussure. Lévi-Strauss broadens systems of differences from signs as words to a wider context of signs as myths, as well as social structures and patterns of relation; Lévi-Strauss' specific cross-cultural accounts of diametric and concentric space concerning social structures and myths are broadened to other systems of relation, including language and elsewhere (Downes 2012, 2013) intrapsychic systems of the unconscious. Lévi-Strauss tended to consider diametric and concentric relations as structures, with less emphasis being given to their roles as spaces, whether as part of a spatial process of distanciation or otherwise. Yet the argument for this expanded domain of relevance for diametric and concentric spaces goes beyond simply empirical referents, whether linguistic, psychological or anthropological, and beyond structuralism; it needs to also be an ontological argument for a spatial-phenomenology at the level of primordial structures of being, as a protolanguage for experience.

The system of relations between concentric and diametric spaces offers a spatial discourse of implication independent of language, yet underpinning language in assumed connection with it. In this sense, it is a candidate spatial protolanguage. As the concentric and diametric spatial system of relations precedes the metaphorical as a condition for it, concentric and diametric spaces cannot be reduced to being simply metaphors. As architectures of space constituting pivotal aspects of a protolanguage as a system of meaning through their interactive tension, concentric and diametric spaces offer a more fundamental truth level pertaining to a life system. The issue of a life system in relation to Ricoeur and these spaces is explored in more detail in the final chapter.

An explicit argument is not being made that primordial space operates in a concentric structural relation to language, as manifested in metaphor. Yet the structural resemblances between the differential relations of concentric and diametric space, on the one hand, and metaphor, on the other hand, building on the work of Ricoeur, invite further consideration of this question as a strong possibility.

Notes

1 In Downes (2012), Chapter 8, the Chinese yin/yang symbol is interpreted in terms of primordial spaces of diametric and concentric relation, to highlight the different spatial implications of this discourse in yin/yang from its traditional cultural–historical associations.

2 See Downes (2012), Chapter 9, on the contrasts with Wittgensteinian language games and diametric and concentric spaces, as different levels of description.

3 Ricoeur treats Heidegger's position as 'a laziness in thinking, of lumping the whole of Western thought together under a single word, metaphysics' (MV: 311).

4 Ricoeur offers examples from Fontanier such as 'consuming remorse', 'courage craving for peril and praise', 'the brilliant eagle of Meaux' (MV: 294).

5 See also Derrida on spatial concerns with an entirely other text of a 'new psychoanalytic graphology' to come (1978/1981: 231) and Downes (2013) for an amplification of this.

6 Such a breath–body relation is not a diametric mirror image inversion between both dimensions, it is not a diametric split of assumed separation between breath and body; breath and body need each other, they are mutually entwined. This relation is a 'breath in body–body' phenomenological connection, a concentric spatial relation where the breath is the inner circle for the outer circle of the body (Downes 2012). For another discussion of the breath in relation to being, see also Derrida (1991).

7 Ricoeur also draws on Aquinas' argument that even causality has to be thought of as analogical, where there is some relation of the creature to God as its principle and cause (MV: 277). For an analysis of causality in spatial terms of diametric mirror image symmetry, see Downes (2016). For an account of traces or fragments of the transcendental horizon in the empirical, as the background relation between concentric and diametric spaces, see Downes (2012), Chapter 11.

8 See also Richardson (1974: 74). In *What is Metaphysics?*, Heidegger highlights 'an essential distinction' between 'comprehending the whole of beings as such and finding oneself in the midst of beings as a whole.' The former truth as totality claim is 'impossible in principle' (Heidegger 1929/1993: 99).

9 See Downes (2012) for an argument regarding this dynamic background horizon for concentric and diametric spaces in terms of early Heidegger's transcendental horizon of temporality and non-simple structural whole of care.

10 See Downes (2012) for an account of the roles of concentric and diametric spaces at these different levels of transcendental horizon, horizontal–ontological and ontic referential fragments.

11 The entailments of diametric and concentric spaces in relation to image schemata is interpreted, as follows, in Downes (2010, 2012):

Diametric spatial schema	*Concentric spatial schema*	*Image schema structure*
Assumed separation	Separation on the basis of assumed connection	Containers (interior, boundary, exterior); boundedness, differentiation
Assumed separation and non-interaction between foreground diametric poles and background space	Assumed connection and interaction between concentric poles and background space centre–periphery	Foreground–background; part–whole relation; object–location dual
Mirror image inverted symmetry	Symmetry as identity	Contrastive pairs as opposites–inversions

References

D'Aquili, E., 'The Influence of Jung on the Work of Claude Lévi-Strauss'', *Journal of the History of the Behavioral Sciences*, 1975, 11: 41–48.

Derrida, J., *The Ear of the Other: Otobiography, Transference, Translation*. C. V. MacDonald (ed.), trans. P. Kamuf. New York: Schocken Books, 1985.

Derrida, J., *Of Spirit: Heidegger and the Question*. Trans. G. Bennington and R. Bowlby. Chicago, IL: University of Chicago Press, 1991.

Derrida, J., *On Touching – Jean-Luc Nancy*. Stanford, CA: Stanford University Press, 2005.

Downes, P., 'Cross-Cultural Structures of Concentric and Diametric Dualism in Lévi-Strauss' Structural Anthropology: Structures of Relation Underlying the Self and Ego Relation?', *Journal of Analytical Psychology*, 2003, 48: 47–81.

Downes, P., *The Primordial Dance: Diametric and Concentric Spaces in the Unconscious World*. Oxford/Bern: Peter Lang, 2012.

Downes, P., 'Developing Derrida's Psychoanalytic Graphology: Diametric and Concentric Spatial Movements', *Derrida Today*, 2013, 6(2): 197–221.

Downes, P., 'Concentric and Diametric Spatial Structures of Relation: Exploring a Neutral Bridge Language Between Quantum Physics and Neuropsychology', *Neuroquantology, An Interdisciplinary Journal of Neuroscience and Quantum Physics*, 2016, 14(3): 885.

Grünbaum, A., 'Précis of 'The Foundations of Psychoanalysis: A Philosophical Critique'', *Behavioral and Brain Sciences*, 1986, 9: 217–284.

Habermas, J., *Knowledge and Human Interests*. Cambridge: Polity Press, 1972/2007.

Heidegger, M., *What is Metaphysics?*, in D. F. Krell (ed.), *Basic Writings*. New York: HarperCollins, 1929/1993.

Jakobson, R., 'Results of the Conference of Anthropologists and Linguists', in *Selected Writings II: Word and Language*. Paris/The Hague: Mouton, 1971.

Körner, S., 'The Impossibility of Transcendental Deductions', *Monist*, 1967, 51: 317–331.

Lakoff, G. and Johnson, M., *Philosophy in the Flesh: The Embodied Mind and its Challenge to Western Thought*. New York: Basic Books, 1999.

Lewis, I. M., 'Introduction', in I. M. Lewis (ed.), *Symbols and Sentiments: Cross-Cultural Studies in Symbolism*. London: Academic Press, 1977.

Richardson, W. J., *Through Phenomenology to Thought*, 3rd ed. The Hague: Martinus Nijhoff, 1974.

Chapter 10

Space and internalisation of the other

A living spatial movement of relation – reconceptualising life in spatial terms in Ricoeur's Oneself as another via Heidegger's *Being and Time*

In *Oneself as Another*, Ricoeur confronts the dismantling of a static and monolithic human subject, such as that of the Cartesian selfgrounding *cogito*. Ricoeur seeks a divided and dynamic subjectivity. This 'dividing line' (OA: 318) that he excavates runs across the crevice between self as sameness (*idem*) and self as oneself (*ipse*), which he views as two fundamental modes of being, in a dynamic dialectical tension that evades any simple appeal to foundations. This dividing line opens up a gateway beyond a univocal self to a wider questioning, with an array of intertwining strands of argument, in quest of these two purportedly fundamental modes of being, dynamically interacting.

Key strands of Ricoeur's argument involve search for a constituting structure of the other in the self, not as external to self. Allied with this is a concern to bridge the cavern between Heidegger's *Dasein* and an acting self as subjectivity. Both of these strands pertain to life principles either directly or indirectly apprehended by Ricoeur. Search for a constituting structure of the other in the self is a question already raised in terms of a life principle by Dilthey, although as early Heidegger observes, it remained unanswered by Dilthey (Heidegger 2009: 254).[1]

Ricoeur's engagement with a life dimension for this constituting structure of the other takes place more directly as part of a life and wellbeing concern with 'living well with and for others' (OA: 330). Ricoeur's bridging principle between Heidegger's *Dasein* and the self as acting subject is derived from Spinoza's *conatus* as power to act, and again expressly related by Ricoeur to life, to life as power. His discussion of *conatus* and the power to act is in terms of 'the internal dynamism worthy of the name life' linked with power: '[I]t is in man that *conatus*, or the power of being of all things, is most clearly readable'(OA: 316); Ricoeur sees power and life as interchangeable, 'the power or life', 'this power of animation', when summarising Spinoza approvingly (OA: 316–317).

When Ricoeur seeks to associate if not equate *conatus* as power to act with Heidegger's care – a core structure of *Dasein* – it is tempting to treat both as held together through the common connection of a life principle, given that early Heidegger (2009) also expressly treated care as pivotal to life.[2]

Beyond the disparate and mainly fleeting references to life in Ricoeur's *Oneself as Another*, whether as life as power, living well and with others, factical life, as well as Ricoeur's attempt to develop a concept of embodied subjectivity as flesh that is presumably living flesh, not dead flesh, a further and arguably primordial life principle needs to be brought to the fore, namely, *living space*. How does this proposed living space appear as a dynamic phenomenon? Ricoeur engages with this question although not directly in such words or terms.

A significant conceptual leap takes place in Ricoeur's later work (*OA*), a leap that is embedded in the seeds of *La Métaphore Vive* but ultimately resting simply as a promissory note in that work.[3] This leap forward is Ricoeur's recognition of the vital significance of space primordially, as a pivotal dimension that is even *prior* to language. His search in this latter work is for a prelinguistic primordial spatial structure to give expression to, or at least to lay bare, the relation between self and other. Ricoeur recognises that: 'On the basis of the model of the problem of localizing the flesh, other problems relating to the primordial spatiality of the flesh could be posed ... As Jean-Luc Petit has established ... it is upon this *prelinguistic* relation between my flesh localized by the self and a world accessible or inaccessible to the "I can" that a semantics of action is finally to be constructed which will not lose its way in the endless exchange of language games' (OA: 325) (emphasis added).

Continuing on this theme of spatialisation, Ricoeur asks: 'We may wonder if the phenomenology of spatiality, so propitiously begun in Husserl, receives the attention it deserves in Heidegger' (OA: 328). This acceleration of focus on space in later Ricoeur contrasts somewhat with MV, where spatial understandings also pervade much of Ricoeur's discussion of metaphor in terms of proximity and distance, tension, substitution, displacement, change of location, image, the 'open' structure of words, closure, transparency and opaqueness. Yet, as argued in the previous chapter, this is usually where space is discussed within metaphor, and as a metaphor itself, rather than as a precondition or prior system of relations to language interacting with language.

A living space as a dynamic interacting background is in stark contrast with a Cartesian conception of space as 'empty' and a 'mere nonentity' (Descartes 1954: 200). The nuanced position of Ricoeur is not simply that he recognises that the Heidegger of *Being and Time* gives limited although notable attention to space; it is that Ricoeur quests for a space that avoids the Scylla of reduction to geometric or 'objective' space and the Charybdis of *collapsing the subtlety of space into mere place*. A spatial turn is increasingly recognised across the social sciences[4] aided and abetted by commentators on Heidegger[5] that aptly emphasise the central importance of space in *Being and Time* and elsewhere in

Heidegger's work. However, commentators on Heidegger's spatial understanding, such as Elden and Malpas, then flatten the dimensionality that space offers conceptually into a scrutiny of space simply as location, as mere places, as part of a sociohistorical critique of space. The significance of Ricoeur's exploration in OA is that he amplifies space in search of an ontology of space and in doing so, he does not engage in an *écrasement* of space into place.

Whereas space moves forward in Ricoeur's OA, to take a centre stage as a foregrounded concept for interrogation, a life principle or movement nevertheless remains held together in the background fabric of the assumptions of his work on selfhood as a living power to act. The role of a life principle here is pervasive if not omnipresent as Ricoeur is still rejecting, in Heideggerian vein, a substance ontology of *ousia* as presence, and especially its Latin version as *substantia*.

The main argument of this chapter is that a spatial-phenomenology and ontology is possible, and that Ricoeur stepped towards this before diverting into a Husserlian retreat, via an ontology of the flesh. The concern for current purposes is less to subdue the Husserlian emphasis of Ricoeur but to highlight an alternative pathway in *Being and Time* for Ricoeur's bridging mode between *Dasein* and subjectivity, as a primordial spatiality. Implications for understanding the relation between *conatus* and care, as dimensions of a living space principle will be examined. The proposed primordial spatial discourse of concentric and diametric space will also be proposed to elucidate Ricoeur's key concern with a structure, a mediating structure between self and other, what he terms the metacategory of otherness. This issue of a mediating structure between self and other, whether one of inclusion or exclusion, is a preoccupation shared with both Schopenhauer and Nietzsche, as explored in Chapter 3 regarding compassion.

Beyond Lévi-Strauss' structuralism to the interplay between diametric and concentric spaces as pure spatial movement in Heidegger's *Being and Time*

Ricoeur comments on Heidegger that 'the spatial dimension of being-in-the-world appears to involve mainly the inauthentic forms of care ... We may then wonder if it is not the unfolding of the problematic of temporality, triumphant in the second section of *Being and Time*, that prevented an *authentic* phenomenology of spatiality' (OA: 328). Ricoeur's proposed ontology of the flesh is one dimension towards expression of an authentic phenomenology of spatiality, *although not necessarily the only one*. There may be other pathways towards a fundamental ontology and phenomenology of space.

Ricoeur seeks to carve out a conceptual domain with strong affinity with Heidegger – a domain of truth prior to apophantic judgment of Aristotle, that is not committed to a substance ontology. Ricoeur rejects Aristotle's 'presumed pre-eminence of assertive judgment, of apophansis' of being-true and being-false as a basis for attestation as certainty (of continuity of self as *idem*). In doing so, Ricoeur is firmly within Heidegger's similar distancing from apophantic truth of Aristotle in his search for a primordial truth domain. Ricoeur's recognition of the 'difficulty' of Aristotle's 'primacy of actuality over potentiality in connection with the theory of substance' (OA: 306) is again firmly in Heidegger's territory of *Being and Time*. Yet Ricoeur goes even further and aspires to a structural affinity between the role key concepts of Heidegger play in his architecture of being and Ricoeur's own architecture of selfhood. Thus, Heidegger's conscience is resonant with Ricoeur's attestation, self as sameness with Heidegger's being present at hand (*Vorhandenheit*), and care with *conatus* as power to act.

There is significant nuance in Ricoeur's accelerated preoccupation with space, as primordial spatiality, and in his recognition of the need to counterbalance Heidegger's prioritising of time, of temporality as the transcendental horizon for the question of being in *Being and Time*. The counterbalance proffered by Ricoeur is of primordial spatiality. Early Heidegger describes time as a pure movement. Heidegger's early Aristotle lectures recognise that: 'The being of life is seen as the movement that has run its courses within itself, in this life … the being of life itself has to be regarded solely in terms of such a movement of pure temporalization … in its genuine movement when it has given up every kind of concern for practical orientation and apprehends simply' (Heidegger 2009a: 176). The current argument is for life as a movement of pure spatialisation, a movement of concentric and diametric spaces that has given up every kind of concern for practical orientation and is a mode of self-propagation. It is being sought to develop space as pure movement, as a dimension of a primordial life principle. Space is examined as a pure living movement as a relation, not substance. Concentric and diametric space invite understanding of space as pure movement, a pure movement of relative differences.

Ricoeur comments on French structuralism in general:

> [T]he *linguistic turn* … has often signified a refusal to 'go outside' of language and a mistrust equal to that of French structuralism with respect to any extralinguistic order … the implicit axiom that everything is language has often led to a closed semanticism, incapable of accounting for human action as actually happening in the world … a phenomenology like Husserl's, according to which the stratum of language is ineffectual in relation to the life of intentional consciousness, has a corrective value, just because it proposes the opposite extreme. (OA: 301)

Ricoeur signals some distance from the linguistic turn. He displays on openness to a level prior to or, at least, beyond language, while situating French structuralism and hence Lévi-Strauss, as locked with linguistic assumptions, although overlooking that his concentric and diametric structural relations were in some way prior to language; this feature of concentric and diametric relations being prior to language was, however, not emphasised by Lévi-Strauss. It would seem that Lévi-Strauss overlooked concentric and diametric structures as a discourse fundamentally of space due to his own structuralist commitments to the primacy of language.

As relative *a priori* entailments, the relative differences between concentric and diametric spaces have in previous chapters been firmly distinguished from Lévi-Strauss' structuralist anthropology and its empirical objectivist paradigm, drawn from phonetics invoking structures as communication. This is not to deny some commonalities between Lévi-Strauss' structuralism and Heidegger, such as search for transsubjective background relations prior to causality and intentionality.[6]

It is being argued that while Ricoeur has acutely perceived the importance of key issues regarding an ontology of space, a dialectical structure for two modes of being, a structure of self that includes otherness in its constitution, the way that he has addressed them needs to move along a somewhat different path than that he traversed in OA. Put simply, in response to the fundamental question of a selfhood made flesh, an embodied dimension of self to provide the sustenance of continuity for the self as same, as *idem*, Ricoeur turns away from Heidegger and towards Husserl, while still recognising that this quest must not fall into the *cogito*-related comforts of representation, of intentionality. Ricoeur views Husserl rather than Heidegger's *Being and Time* as closer to an ontology of the flesh. Yet Ricoeur could have developed a different path, namely, of following through further on spatiality in Heidegger as a pathway to a selfhood, through concentric and diametric primordial spaces of relation. This spatial-phenomenological interpretation of *Being and Time* goes further than engagement with Heidegger's explicit spatial themes to unthought spatial structures (prior to space treated simply as a metaphor) pervading a wider range of its key concepts.[7]

Focus for current purposes is on the relation of concentric and diametric spaces to existential spatiality, as well as aspects of *Angst* and care. Resonant with Ricoeur's concerns to interrogate the as-structure of being-as, and belonging-as with regard to the copula as a background dimension to understanding metaphor, for Heidegger: '[B]eing alongside the world … is an *existentiale* founded upon being-in. In these analyses the issue is one of *seeing* a primordial structure of Dasein's being – a structure in accordance with whose phenomenal content the concepts of being must be articulated' (Heidegger 1927: 81, italics in original). This seeing is a phenomenological disclosure that includes sight but is not simply reducible to the visual (Heidegger 1927: 48). In the words of Henrich:

> When abstracting from the richness of phenomenological analyses and focusing solely on the scaffolding of the progression of thought in *Being and Time*, one immediately recognizes that its driving force is the question concerning the unitary structure of the original totality of Dasein … Yet how is this concept of the ontological structural unity of Dasein different from the speculative interpretations of subjectivity? (1994: 48)

For early Heidegger, there is a primordial structural totality of being-in-the-world, prior to predicative assertion, that encompasses *Dasein*'s spatial structures but somehow extends beyond them; it is less a process of abstracting structures than uncovering them in their surreptitious immanence. Primordial structures of being-in-the-world are irreducible to derivative subjective unconscious structures. Heidegger's purportedly primordial structures of relation include 'being-alongside' as 'being-in', both modes 'equiprimordial' with 'being-with' (1927: 187).

Much of Heidegger's argument in BT rests on the uncovering of a set of structures, where some aspects are treated as prior to others, through a series of relations in a structural whole – a structural whole that was itself never quite manifested as a concrete spatial projection. In the absence of a clearly visualised spatial structure or holistic set of structures, much of Heidegger's account falls away into an argument merely by authority.[8]

It is clear that Heidegger sought in *Being and Time* to uncover specific, concrete, *a priori* spatial ontological structures and did not succeed in doing so. His project lies incomplete. Filling this vacuum for interpretation of Heidegger has brought importation of a Wittgensteinian schema of shared background practices onto background contexts of being in the work of Guignon (1983, 2006), Dreyfus (1991), as well as Malpas (2008), while Malpas has also sought to interpret Heidegger through an Aristotelian schema of spatial containment as *topos*.

Spatiality of being-in-the-world is expressly linked in Division One, III, 21c of *Being and Time* with the earlier discussions of being-in and the two modes of 'categories' and *existentialia*. Seeking to transcend the nature–culture binary opposition in his conceptualisation of space, Heidegger develops these contrasting modes of spatial relation. Traditional Western conceptions of 'world' oversimplify this existential conception of being-in. Being-in, as a *category*, is like water in a glass or a dress in a closet, whereas the *existential* mode of being-in-the-world is a different spatial mode of being-in, which overcomes a distance or remoteness within the categorial mode of being-in. Existential remoteness is not something measurable in terms of objective spatial distances of objectively present entities, as Heidegger explicates, in a well-known passage:

> 'The table stands "by" ["*be*"] the door' or 'the chair "touches" ["*berührt*"] the wall'. Taken strictly, 'touching' is never what we are talking about in such cases, not because accurate reexamination will always eventually establish that there is a space between the chair and the wall, but because in principle the chair can never touch the wall, even if the space between them should be equal to zero. If the chair could touch the wall, this would presuppose that the wall is the sort of thing 'for' which a chair would be encounterable. An entity present-at-hand within the world can be touched by another entity only if by its very nature the latter entity has being-in as its own kind of being. (1927: 81–82)

Relations between solid objects in space are diametric, as there is a basic assumed separation between each object as an object. Both objects exclude each other from occupying the same space. This assumed separation means they are not 'encounterable'; encountering overcomes the remoteness of assumed separation and is a concentric possibility that *Dasein* as being-in-the-world possesses. Heidegger explicitly equates the 'touch' of encountering with the mode of being-alongside. For Heidegger, entities such as a table, chair cannot even *potentially* be encounterable. Against this backdrop, it is notable that Ricoeur refers to 'primordial features' such as touch (OA: 324).

Heidegger challenges the primacy of 'side-by-side-ness' or the separation built into two entities in order for them to be 'side-by-side'. He overcomes a diametric relation between *Dasein*, being and 'world' in his description of 'being-alongside' the world: 'There is no such thing as the "side-by-side-ness" of an entity called "Dasein" with another entity called "world"' (1927: 81). *Diametric space is where both parts are side-by-side.* Heidegger seeks to go beyond Cartesian separation between self and world – beyond a diametric split structure of relation between self and world, subject and object.

In contrast to diametric structured space as side-by-sideness, Heidegger interrogates a different spatial relation of dwelling 'alongside'. For a mode of 'being-alongside' the world, a different mode of assumed connection is needed, which is not a diametric 'side-by-side' relation. Concentric space expresses a 'being-alongside' model of relatedness, where one pole dwells within and alongside the other, surrounded and in assumed connection. The smaller, inner pole within concentric space is far from being a mere bungalow annex to the larger pole. Rather it dwells centrally within the other larger pole, immersed within it inextricably, in complementary fashion as a primordial belonging. Concentric spatialisation offers an existential structural relation that overcomes the remoteness and non-involvement within diametric space. Furthermore, it offers a spatial relation, where one pole is 'in' the other and, hence, is a being-in. Being-alongside is founded on being-in for Heidegger.[9] It is *movement between* contrasting spaces of diametric 'side-by-side' and concentric 'alongside' structures of relation that offers a framework for primordial spaces as an interactive dance.

De-severance is central to this being-alongside and '*Dasein is essentially de-severance – that is, it is spatial*' (1927: 143, italics in original). A recurrent spatial theme within *Being and Time* is the tension between loss of interactive relation and an overcoming of this loss. Some typical examples of this tension between two modes, an interactive, connective, involved mode and a detached, severed, non-relational mode, respectively, occur in the context of the purported spatiality of being-in-the-world. Heidegger refers to the relational state of de-severance: '"De-severing" amounts to making the farness vanish – that is, making the remoteness of something disappear' (1927: 139). This is thoroughly consistent with a movement from a mode of assumed separation or severance within diametric structures of relation, to a spatial mode of assumed connection summoning concentric structures of relation: '*The circumspective de-severing of*

Dasein's everydayness reveals the being-in-itself of the "true world" – of that entity which Dasein, as something existing, is already alongside' (1927: 141, italics in original). Being-in gives expression to the 'true' authentic world of its existential space through de-severance, which brings a return to an already being-alongside, to a concentric assumed connection.

As a feature together with the 'directionality' of the spatiality of being-in-the-world (1927: 138), Heidegger treats de-severance as movement towards a more connective state: 'Every bringing-close has already taken in advance a direction towards a region out of which what is de-severed brings itself close' (1927: 143). This connective state of de-severing reveals a being already alongside (1927: 141). Loss of interactive relation is highlighted in Heidegger's words: 'The spatiality of what is ready-to-hand within-the-world loses its involvement character ... the world loses its specific aroundness' (1927: 147). In concentric space, the outer pole surrounds or is 'around' the inner pole, a feature lost to diametric space; in concentric relation, one part is always 'in' the other, unlike diametric relation. A concentric structure is a mode of being-in, and, for Heidegger: 'Being-in is not a "property" which Dasein sometimes has and sometimes does not have' (1927: 84); it is a fundamental feature of *Dasein*'s existence. The inner concentric circle is interpretable as being in a mode of 'being-in' the outer. The 'spatially encountered' (1927: 143) being-alongside is a concernful, connective (de-severant), concentric mode, which is subject to a displacement or falling, where *Dasein* can become 'rid of its being-alongside' (1927: 237). In other words, the concentric being-alongside can be displaced into a diametric relation, where its relation to *Dasein*'s 'ownmost potentiality-for-being is an issue' (1927: 225).

De-severance is an active process of interaction for *Dasein*, who 'cannot wander about with the current range of its de-severances; it can never do more than change them' (1927: 143). *Dasein*'s primordial connective space undoes the assumed separation in its engagement, what Heidegger calls encountering: 'Dasein is spatial in that it discovers space circumspectively, so that indeed it constantly comports itself de-severantly towards the entities thus spatially encountered' (1927: 143). It is evident that for Heidegger an interaction takes place between this primordial spatial relation and that space of entities diametrically side-by-side one another that is, thereby, changed through this interaction, what Heidegger also terms directionality. They are not simply two spaces divided into existential and 'objective' space, spliced from each other, as Dreyfus (1991) envisages. To do so, would be to reimport a subject–object dualism through a kind of subjective versus objective space, very much contrary to the project of Heidegger.

The very distinction of subject–object is challenged by Heidegger in his spatial conception of *Dasein*. In spatial terms, Heidegger is challenging the ineluctability of the potentially malleable diametric structural relation that frames the subject–object relation. Thomson summarises Heidegger's insight into this assumed separation, with implications for a diametric spatial understanding: 'As Heidegger frequently points out, in the modern, post-Cartesian world, an "object", *Gegenstand*, is something that "stands opposite" a human subject, something *external* to subjectivity' (2011: 49). Diametric spatial relation is such a standing opposite, a counterstand; a spatial precondition for objectification is diametric space through its assumed separation and distanciation, where the diametric poles are opposite one another.

This characterisation of existential space as a concentric structure and of extended space as a diametric structure offers a number of advantages over other interpretations (e.g., Dreyfus 1991; Malpas 2008). It provides domains of interaction between both spaces as envisaged by Heidegger. Treating both spaces as part of the ontological structure of being-in-the-world paves the way not only for their interaction but also for a view of them as key to Heidegger's transcendental project – as the relational interaction between *existentialia* and categories is viewed by early Heidegger as key to the transcendental horizon for the question of being: 'The connection between these two modes of the characters of being [*existentialia* and categories] cannot be handled until the horizon for the question of being has been clarified' (1927: 71). While Malpas (2008) does centrally acknowledge the need for uncovering a primordial spatial structure, the specific concrete structures of concentric and diametric spaces go further than simply an assertion of the need for such primordial spatial structures. The interpretation of existential spatiality as a concentric mode of spatial relation and extended space as a diametric mode of spatial relation does not treat Heidegger's spatiality of being-in-the-world as fundamentally confused, in the fashion of Dreyfus (1991: 129).

For Heidegger: 'Dasein takes space in; this is to be understood literally' (1927: 419). The taking in of diametric space into *Dasein*'s existential spatiality is a more radical step than simply movement towards a concentric space; it is a restructuring, a modification of the diametric space, so that it is taken in by or dissolved into the concentric holistic space. Insofar as diametric space is engaged with 'objective' extended space, its being-taken-in through interaction with concentric space becomes a process of literal change to this relation in extended space. The interaction with concentric structured space brings literal effects in extended space, influences mediated through concentric spatial openings.

Existential spatiality of *Dasein*'s being-in is a concentric spatial structure of assumed connection. *Dasein*'s existential spatiality is a dynamic process of taking space in, it is a directional movement towards concentric structured space. This concentric directional movement belongs to being-in and its equiprimordial dimensions of being-alongside and being-with that involve directionality and de-severance. All are part of the same concentric spatial movement.

Care and *conatus*, *Angst* and suffering

Dissociating the notion of existence from substance and instead relating it to the act, Ricoeur regards the body as a 'nonrepresentative certainty' (OA: 321) involving resistance that gives way to effort, thereby, echoing Maine de Biran explicitly and, more implicitly a Nietzschean concern in BT with pre-representative experience of the Dionysian apprehension of music. A notable feature of Ricoeur's account is a bridging concept between *Dasein* and selfhood as *idem*, as continuity through a structure of *conatus* akin to Heideggerian care; this bridging concept requires an affective dimension, and Ricoeur supplies this sentience for *conatus* as the power to act, namely, through the addendum to *conatus* of suffering.

Ricoeur seeks to develop a bridge in spatial terms between Heidegger's *Dasein* and subjectivity. While pursuing this task, he develops a parallel between Heidegger's care and a conception of *conatus* as power to act and within this emphasises a key dimension of suffering that offers at least indirect parallels with Heidegger's *Angst* as a key structural element of care. Flesh for Ricoeur is 'this original correlation between acting and suffering' (OA: 320); Ricoeur seeks 'a sharp edged dialectic between praxis and pathos' (OA: 320), along an axis resonant with Heidegger's care–*Angst* entwinement.

Ricoeur treats *conatus* as a response to his concern with continuity of self, of self as *idem*, 'the idea of *conatus* stands out, as the effort to persevere in being, which forms the unity of man as of every individual' (OA: 316). From this vantage point, Heideggerian care is being reinterpreted in Ricoeurean terms as a key dimension to continuity of selfhood, to self as *idem*.[10] Sameness of self is for Ricoeur related to Heidegger's *Vorhandenheit* – presence at hand. Flesh can be construed as a softening of a rigid diametric side-by-sideness between separate bodies. Yet a discourse of living spatial movements in terms of concentric and diametric spaces can be further developed with regard to Heidegger's key concepts of *Angst* and care, as fundamental influences on Ricoeur's whole framework, to further concretise Ricoeur's search in spatial phenomenological and ontological terms.

On this proposed reading of early Heidegger's conceptions of encountering and being-alongside, as projections of concentric existential structures in contrast with diametric structures, *Angst* can be examined as the process of openness to movement – of openness to change from and between concentric and diametric spatial modes of relation structuring experience. For Heidegger: 'The turning away of falling is grounded rather in anxiety, which in turn is what first makes fear possible' (1927: 230). Diametric structures involve a turning away from concentric spatialisation. This turning away uncovers the dynamic compensatory interaction between concentric and diametric structures of experience, mediated through *Angst*. Similarly, being-alongside undergoes a 'falling', which again illustrates this directional movement, as the being-alongside of concentric spatialisation turns away towards a diametric mode. *Angst*, as the dynamic component of change and movement between concentric and diametric spaces, brings a focus on change and transformation within experience; this can take place in concentric modes of encountering and being-alongside. These primordial structures also encompass a falling, fleeing, turning away dimension into inauthenticity, as a direction towards diametric space. This structural interplay explains how inauthenticity can still be a *primordial* state of relation; falling, fleeing inauthenticity is implicated in its directional movement away from concentric structures and towards diametric space. Heidegger observes the possibility of *Dasein* 'becoming ... rid of its being alongside' (1927: 216), so that a radical shift from concentric to diametric structures would occur.

Angst invokes a futural direction of possible movement towards authentic concentric spatialisation, through modifying diametric structures – through modifying a state of assumed separation into a state of separation on the basis of assumed connection. This sense of directional movement, towards the 'aroundness' of concentric relation, gains indirect support from Christenson's examination of the translation of Heidegger's understanding of purpose, in his phrase '*etwas, um zu*'. While MacQuarrie and Robinson (1962: 98) note the dual meaning of *um* as 'around' and 'in order to', Christenson amplifies this point:

> The German phrase *etwas, um zu* ..., which MacQuarrie and Robinson translate as 'something-in-order-to', is, while not ungrammatical, certainly unusual; one would normally speak of *etwas zum*, as in *etwas zum schreiben*, i.e., something for writing. This indicates that Heidegger is placing weight on what the expressions in the phrase individually mean. In particular, he is placing weight on the meaning of the word *um*. In German this word doubles as a preposition meaning 'around', as in *um die Ecke* ('around the corner') and as a prefix meaning 'surrounding', as in *Umwelt*. (2007: 165)

A key distinguishing feature of concentric from diametric space is that, in the former, the outer pole 'surrounds' and is 'around' the inner, in a relation of assumed connection – a dimension that is not obtainable in diametric relation. Purpose, envisaged as directional change towards concentric spatialisation of surrounding and being around, is thus consistent with Christenson's conclusion, regarding Heidegger's emphasis on '*um*': 'It is thus reasonable to conclude that Heidegger is using the unusual phrase *etwas, um zu* ... in order to exploit, on the one hand, the meaning of the whole phrase *um-zu* as expressing purpose, and, on the other, the meaning of the component word *um* as expressing aroundness' (2007: 165). Concentric spatial projection is a directional movement towards aroundness.

Interpreting care, Ricoeur recognises that: 'Everything turns, as we know, on the sense of the preposition "in", which has not equivalent on the side of the relation among beings belong to the metacategory of *Vorhandenheit*' (OA: 310). For early Heidegger, both care and primordial temporality must be interpreted in structural terms: '[T]he care-structure does not speak against the possibility of being-a-whole but is the condition for the possibility' of this potentiality (1927: 365). For Heidegger, the care structure is not simple, although it is central to the question of the unity of the structural whole of *Dasein*, as 'Dasein can be spatial only as care' (1927: 419). Care embraces the contours and structures of *Dasein*'s existential spatiality, but goes further.

While the interplay between care and primordial temporality in relation to a proposed primordial spatial discourse of concentric and diametric spaces is explored in more detail elsewhere (Downes 2012), suffice for current purposes to outline this argument in preliminary terms. A further dimension interrogated in this spatial-phenomenological reading of *Being and Time* focuses on the background relation *itself* between concentric and diametric spaces, to go beyond treating these spaces in diametric fashion as operating 'side-by-side' to one another. Heidegger's inquiry into 'the meaning of care' asks 'what makes possible the totality of the articulated structural whole of care' (1927: 371). Is there a background relation engaging with the structure of care? This focus on a more primordial dimension than concentric (authentic) and diametric (inauthentic) spaces invites a questioning of the background spatial relation *itself between* concentric and diametric spaces. Is this background spatial relation between concentric and diametric spaces itself a concentric one of assumed connection or a diametric one of assumed separation?

A diametric spatial relation between concentric and diametric spaces would be a split between both spaces to minimise their interaction. The connective feature of care is a background spatial movement of concentric spatial direction towards unifying the foreground spatial structures of concentric and diametric spaces. However, this background is in an ongoing dynamic tension between a connective care as a concentric spatial direction, on the one hand, and an assumed separation, a diametric split in the background itself between concentric and diametric spaces, on the other. The direction of connective concentric care, as a background relation between *Dasein*'s concentric and diametric structures of existence, is not static; neither is it the only possible direction. Care encompasses both the background connective relation between *Dasein*'s concentric and diametric structures and these structures of *Dasein* themselves; it becomes *both connective background and the totality of the foreground spatial structures.*[11]

Although care expresses concentric structured authenticity, the contrary space of diametric inauthenticity is made visible as a potential structure. Like *Angst*, care includes an awareness of the potential for movement between authenticity and inauthenticity, between concentric and diametric spaces. However, care goes further than *Angst* to a prior connective directional level. For this possibility of movement between concentric and diametric spaces, a prior background temporal dimension is a necessary condition; in Heidegger's words: '*Temporality reveals itself as the meaning of authentic care … the primordial unity of the structure of care lies in temporality*' (1927: 374–375, italics in original).

Yet the intrusion of *conatus* as a kind of Heideggerian care, to bridge an ontological chasm between Heidegger's *Dasein* and Ricoeur's selfhood as continuity of self, as *idem*, brings with it a commitment to power. Ricoeur cites Spinoza: '[T]he power or *conatus* by which it perseveres in its own being, is nothing but the given, or actual essence of the thing, p.110' (OA: 316).

Power (to act) imports a diametric spatial relation. This is an implication of another feature of diametric space, mirror image inverted symmetry. Diametric mirror image symmetry is a spatial precondition for mirror image oppositions framing power relations, such as between upper–lower, superior–inferior, master–slave, powerful–powerless. The concentric assumed connection of care becomes twisted into a diametric power realm that necessarily brings a power hierarchy. It is resonant with the twist within Nietzsche's work where the will to life becomes inverted into a mirror image opposition as will to power.

Regarding Nietzsche's good and bad conscience in GM, Ricoeur highlights 'a problem in Nietzsche to determine whether the reference, assured by the genealogical method, to "strong" or "weak" Life, reaches the ultimate referent of a terminal deciphering' (OA: 345). What Ricoeur hints at here is the displacement from the diametric mirror image symmetry of good–bad conscience to strong–weak life of a master–slave morality as remaining locked with a diametric spatial frame of reference that is far from being a fundamental resolution of this issue. Again Nietzsche's creditor–debtor account of morals as an owing is a frame in terms of diametric mirror image symmetries. Ricoeur observes the 'authoritarian tone' (OA: 346) of Nietzsche's claim to have discovered the 'origin' of the moral conceptual world. When Ricoeur criticises the 'new dogmatism' of Nietzsche where 'all the reversals made by the genealogical method [are] being intended to destroy teleology with the weapons of archaeology' (OA: 346), he could go further through the realisation that Nietzsche is projecting here a distinctive space as will to power, a quasi-compulsive repetition of diametric space as mirror image inversions and that this is not the only possible experiential space for understanding conscience.

A further key diametric mirror image reversal relied on by Ricoeur in his account of suffering underlying *conatus* as the bridge between *Dasein* and subjectivity, is that of active–passive: '[T]he basic dissymmetry, inherent in interaction, resulting from the fact that an agent, by exerting a power over another, treats the latter as the patient of his or her action' (OA: 320). Ricoeur here engages in an explicit appeal to issues of symmetry. However, this active–passive inversion is not dissymmetry but mirror image inverted symmetry.

Ricoeur's *conatus* as power to act interrogates power as a reigning: 'Starting from this otherness, I can reign over. Primordiality, however, is not a reign. Ontologically, the flesh precedes the distinction between the voluntary and the involuntary' (OA: 324). On a spatial-phenomenological reading in terms of concentric and diametric spaces, Ricoeur is treating the diametric power dimension of a reign as not being primordial. However, this may be a conflation of the authentic and the primordial. On a reading of *Being and Time* in terms of concentric and diametric spaces as care, the diametric space is primordial but inauthentic – and, for Heidegger, the inauthentic can still be primordial and requires a structural modification to be authentic. A further problem here with Ricoeur's position is the invocation of power dimensions solely to subjective will as voluntary–involuntary. In contrast, diametric spatial systems of relation propagate themselves prior to simply subjective will and hence the power force in diametric space is more akin to Nietzsche's impersonal will to power as a system of self-propagating diametric spaces. Ricoeur's quest for an '*authentic* phenomenology of spatiality' (OA: 328) needs to disaggregate the primordial–derivative and authentic–inauthentic axes.

Ricoeur seeks a power relation that is not one of sheer diametric space of master–slave: 'And what are we to say of the Other when he is the executioner? And who will be able to distinguish the master from the executioner, the master who calls for a disciple from the master who requires a slave?' interrogates 'reciprocity ... in which the roles are continually reversed' (OA: 339). However, reciprocity as diametric mirror image reversal and inversion requires distinction from reciprocity as assumed connection, of an affective mutual attunement. The glue holding together words such as reciprocity must be stripped bare in spatial terms to reveal fundamental differences of relation.

Care is interpreted as embracing a concentric spatial structure, in stark contrast to the diametric spatial hierarchy of power, whether as the power to act of *conatus* as a living principle or the will to power as a turning within or of the will to life in Nietzsche. This conclusion is not that Heidegger's care and Ricoeur's *conatus* are thus, incommensurable discourses and that Ricoeur's attempt to connect them conceptually is flawed. Rather the opposite is the case. While concentric and diametric spaces are contrasting systems of relation, so that there is a turn and falling in the shift from concentric spatial care to diametric spatial preconditions for power as *conatus* – nevertheless, both are primordial spaces. Both concentric and diametric spaces as structures of relation are themselves in mutual relation; they offer a common discourse of mutual interplay and tension. Hence, in the sense that both concentric care and diametric *conatus* share a primordial spatial discourse, Ricoeur's observation is justified that there is a conceptual transferability from Heidegger's care as a fundamental structure of *Dasein* and *conatus* as a fundamental structure of selfhood in its continuity as a power to act. They play similar roles in a comparable overall architecture or network of mutual relations, even though care is a concentric spatial structure and *conatus* presupposes diametric spatial preconditions. Moreover, care's extra role as background (as well as foreground) connection encompasses the diametric within which *conatus* lurks.

Diametric space as assumed separation and closure: a discourse anticipated by Ricoeur

Selfhood with otherness is explicitly envisaged by Ricoeur as existing in structural terms ('the specific dialectical structure of the relation between selfhood and otherness' (OA: 298)). This dialectic with otherness is an internalisation of the other, which Ricoeur treats as a 'metacategory of otherness' (OA: 298).

The other is in some way a dimension of the primordial structures of self, of relations embedded in the self: 'The fact that otherness is not added on to selfhood from outside, as thought to prevent its solipsistic drift, but that it belongs instead to the tenor of meaning and to the ontological constitution of selfhood' (OA: 317). Ricoeur develops this in OA in three ways: otherness as the body or flesh, otherness as the foreign and the relation of self to itself as conscience.

Ricoeur explores the crevices of the disjunction between Aristotle's actual–potential dimensions of being and a conception of the being of the categories as *ousia*, in order to uncover a space to interrogate the question of the continuity of being in the self as *idem*; paradoxically, he seeks continuity of self through a conceptual device of exploration of disjunction. For his exploration of self in relation to inclusion of the other, he operates a reverse conceptual trajectory, namely, his is a search for a continuity of relation rather than a rupture of an outside, in the relation of self to another.

Ricoeur seeks to strip away the layers of foreignness in the understanding of the other as a constituting relational structure of the self, a foreignness he construes in terms of passivity. A pivotal thread to this foreignness in the structure of the self is that of Heidegger's 'they self', as inauthenticity, a structure requiring modification to turn it towards authenticity. According to Ricoeur, in *Being and Time*: 'Heidegger described perfectly this moment of otherness that distinguishes conscience. Far from being foreign to the constitution of selfhood, this otherness is closely related to its emergence, inasmuch as, under the impetus of conscience, the self is made capable of taking hold of itself in the anonymity of the "they" ... how does the self free itself from the "they"?' (OA: 342).

The anxiety of authenticity reveals the possibility of moving from diametric structures (a category mode of experience) in a direction towards concentric space. From this perspective, authenticity occurs in the modification of diametric structures of experience towards concentric, existential 'being-in' structures. In Heidegger's words: 'Authentic being-one's-self does not rest upon an exceptional condition of the subject, a condition that has been detached from the "they"; it is rather an existentiell modification of the "they" – of the "they" as an essential existentiale' (1927: 168). Heidegger's authentic self, which is not detached or floating above the inauthentic self, can still retain a realm distinct from inauthenticity if the relation is viewed in terms of a concentric relation, where the authentic is the inner circle surrounded by and immersed in the outer inauthentic pole, yet still differentiated from it.

Another entailment of the relative differences between concentric and diametric spaces is foreground–background interaction versus noninteraction. As the concentric poles are in assumed connection to one another, they are also in assumed connection to the background; and this assumed connection to the background resists closure within the concentric structure. Diametric structures' relation to their own poles is one of a mirror image division, which then maintains a cleavage from the background that becomes closed off.

Ricoeur's challenge to a view of interiority as being 'determined solely by the desire for retreat and closure' (OA: 339) is a quest for an interiority that goes beyond diametric spatial closure off of self from other and towards a more open concentric spatial relation. In Ricoeur's words, Husserl's radical selfgrounding 'expresses a will to closure, more precisely a state of separation, that makes otherness the equivalent of radical exteriority' (OA: 335–336); 'separation has made interiority sterile' (OA: 337). Ricoeur explicitly thematises in terms of both closure and separation, key hallmarks of diametric spatial structures relative to concentric space; diametricity is a sterile, inauthentic space for interiority in split opposition to exteriority. Moreover, this thematisation is also explicitly treated in diametric terms if not spatial terms but Ricoeur's recognition that the work of Levinas is 'directed against a conception of the identity of the Same, to which the otherness of the other is diametrically opposed' (OA: 335). From these Ricoeurean threads of a quest for an Otherness that is not closure, separation or diametric opposition, combined with his interrogation of a prelinguistic and primordial spatiality, it is evident that Ricoeur has anticipated a diametric spatial discourse or protolanguage system without naming it as such as a diametric *spatial* structure – and without engaging with its countermovement in explicit spatial terms. This counter-movement needs explicit recognition in terms of a life principle as concentric spatial movements, as inclusion of the Other within part of the identity of the self as a spatial–relational system.

Notes

1 Ricoeur's questioning of a phenomenological and ontological structure of otherness offers strong resonance with a question of life in relation to the other, perhaps best expressed through Heidegger's words on Dilthey: 'Inasmuch as life is life with others, the structures of this life with one another still have to be produced. But how is this life of the other originally given?' (254), a question Heidegger states that Dilthey never pursued further.
2 Heidegger 2009a. Heidegger's Aristotle lectures 'the basic [relational] sense of the movement of factic life is caring [*Sorgen*]' (153). Care is associated for Heidegger with life and movement, movement in the world where: 'The world is there *in* life and *for* life' (155); 'The tendency to lapse is life's evasion of itself … life's own evasion of life and an evasion of life's proper character of being' (158).
3 Downes 2017, 146–163.
4 Gulson and Symes 2007, 97–110; Ferrare and Apple, 2010, 209–221.
5 Elden, 2001; Elden, 2004, 86–105; Malpas, 2008.
6 In *Being and Time*, Heidegger explicitly distinguished his ontological questioning from that of anthropology, due to the latter's subjectivist and ontic, empirical commitments.
7 The interplay between diametric and concentric spaces is argued in Downes, *The Primordial Dance* to be a fundamental implicit feature of Heidegger's *magnum opus*, *Being and Time*, especially, although not exclusively, with regard to the entailments of assumed separation and connection. Concentric and diametric spatial projections are argued to pervade the panorama of Heidegger's basic concepts in *Being and Time* including: (i) *Dasein*'s existential spatiality as being-in, being alongside, directionality, de-severance and encountering, contrasting with the extended space of categories,

(ii) *Angst* of authenticity, (iii) phenomena and appearances, unconcealment (*alethia*), (iv) care as an *a priori* structure and primordial temporality as a transcendental horizon.

8 The poverty of Heidegger's method has been perhaps most forcefully criticised by Ernst Tugendhat (1967). He emphasises the lack of criteria for privileging as primordial in any Heideggerian truth claims, whether for disclosure of being or for preference of a dimension of experience as being authentic.

9 Heidegger, *Being and Time*, 81.

10 Ricoeur recognises that connection between selfhood and *Dasein* is through care for Heidegger: '[T]he most fundamental existential capable of ensuring the thematic unity of the work, at least until temporality appears on the stage in the second section'; *Oneself as Another*, 309.

11 Downes, *The Primordial Dance*. Three distinct levels are argued to emerge in relation to concentric and diametric spatial structures:

i The primordial foreground level of interaction between concentric and diametric spaces, in the *Angst* of *Dasein*'s authenticity and inauthenticity.
ii The prior background level, the phenomenal level prior even to *Dasein*'s existential spatiality. This background level involves, in effect, a selfreferential questioning of whether the relation itself, between concentric and diametric spaces, is a concentric or diametric one. This dynamic, directional tension between the positional structures of concentric and diametric spaces presupposes a temporal dimension.
iii The falling away from primordial spatial structures (of concentric and diametric spaces). The compression, splitting, breaking of the primordial spaces brings them into derivative modes as fragments. This is again a selfreferential process where the foreground fragments emerge from the background direction of a diametric splitting process. This collapse of the primordial structures implicates a different realm of movement and time. It implicates the ontic–historical.

References

Christensen, C. B., 'What are the Categories in Sein und Zeit? Brandom on Heidegger on Zuhandenheit', European Journal of Philosophy, 2007, *15*(*2*): 159–185.

Descartes, R., Descartes: Philosophical writings. Trans. E. Anscombe and P. T. Geach. London: Nelson, 1954.

Downes, P., The Primordial Dance: Diametric and Concentric Spaces in the Unconscious World. Oxford/Bern: Peter Lang, 2012.

Downes, P., 'At the Threshold of Ricoeur's Concerns in La Métaphore Vive: A Spatial Discourse of Diametric and Concentric Structures of Relation Building on Lévi-Strauss', Ricoeur Studies/Etudes Ricoeuriennes, 2017, *7*(*2*): 146–163.

Dreyfus, H. L., Being-in-the World: A Commentary on Heidegger's Being and Time Division I. Cambridge, MA: MIT Press, 1991.

Elden, S., Mapping the present: Heidegger, Foucault and the Project of a Spatial History. London: Continuum, 2001.

Elden, S., 'Between Marx and Heidegger: Politics, philosophy and Lefebvre's "The Production of Space"', Antipode, 2004, *36*: 86–105.

Ferrare, J. J. and Apple, M. W., 'Spatializing Critical Education: Progress and Cautions', Critical Studies in Education, 2010, *51*: 209–221.

Guignon, C. B., Heidegger and the Problem of Knowledge. Indianapolis, IN: Hackett Publishing, 1983.

Guignon, C., 'Authenticity, Moral Values and Psychotherapy', in The Cambridge Companion to Heidegger, 2nd ed.. Cambridge: Cambridge University Press, 2006, 268–292.

Gulson, K. A. and Symes, C., 'Knowing One's Place: Space, Theory, Education', Critical Studies in Education, 2007, *48*: 97–110.

Heidegger, M., 'Wilhelm Dilthey's Research and the Current Struggle for a World-view', in T. Kisiel and T.Sheehan (eds.), *Becoming Heidegger: On the Trail of his Early Occasional Writings 1910–1927*, 2nd revised, expanded ed. Seattle: Noesis Press, 2009.

Heidegger, M., 'Phenomenological Interpretations with Respect to Aristotle: Indication of the Hermeneutical Situation', in T. Kisiel and T.Sheehan (eds.), Becoming Heidegger: On the Trail of his Early Occasional Writings 1910–1927, 2nd revised,expanded ed. Seattle: Noesis Press, 2009a.

Henrich, D., The Unity of Reason: Essays on Kant's Philosophy. Cambridge, MA: Harvard University Press, 1994.

Lévi-Strauss, C., Structural Anthropology, Vol. 1. Trans. C. Jacobsen and B. Grundfest Schoepf. London: Penguin, 1963.

Lévi-Strauss, C., Structural Anthropology, Vol. 2. Trans. M. Layton. London: Penguin Books, 1973/1977.

MacQuarrie, J. and Robinson, E., in *M. Heidegger, Being and Time*, Trans. J. MacQuarrie and E. Robinson. Oxford: Basil Blackwell, 1962.

Malpas, J., Heidegger's Topology: Being, Place, World. Cambridge, MA: MIT Press, 2008.

Thomson, I. D., Heidegger, Art and Modernity. New York: Cambridge University Press, 2011.

Tugendhat, E., Der Wahrheitsbegriff bei Husserl und Heidegger. Berlin: de Gruyter, 1967.

Index

Entries in *italics* refer to figures.

For Product Safety Concerns and Information please contact our EU representative GPSR@taylorandfrancis.com
Taylor & Francis Verlag GmbH, Kaufingerstraße 24, 80331 München, Germany

www.ingramcontent.com/pod-product-compliance
Ingram Content Group UK Ltd.
Pitfield, Milton Keynes, MK11 3LW, UK
UKHW011013180926
475701UK00004B/721
9781032088372